Hypertension
in
Postmenopausal
Women

Hypertension *in* Postmenopausal Women

edited by

Franz H. Messerli

Ochsner Clinic and
Alton Ochsner Medical Foundation
New Orleans, Louisiana

Associate Editor

Franz C. Aepfelbacher

Ochsner Clinic and
Alton Ochsner Medical Foundation
New Orleans, Louisiana

Marcel Dekker, Inc.   New York • Basel • Hong Kong

Library of Congress Cataloging in Publication Data

Hypertension in postmenopausal women / edited by Franz H. Messerli ;
associate editor, Franz C. Aepfelbacher.
    p. cm.
    Includes index.
    ISBN 0-8247-9652-7 (hardcover : alk. paper)
    1. Hypertension in old age. 2. Women--Diseases. 3. Menopause.
4. Menopause--Hormone replacement therapy. I. Messerli, Franz H.
II. Aepfelbacher, Franz C.
    [DNLM: 1. Cardiovascular Diseases--complications.
    2. Postmenopause. 3. Cardiovascular Diseases--in old age.
    4. Hypertension--complications.   WG 120 H998 1996]
    RC685.H8H7853   1996
    616.1'32'00846--dc20
    DNLM/DLC
    for Library of Congress   95-39859
                                                       CIP

The publisher offers discounts on this book when ordered in bulk quantities. For more information, write to Special Sales/Professional Marketing at the address below.

This book is printed on acid-free paper.

Marcel Dekker, Inc.
270 Madison Avenue, New York, New York 10016

Current printing (last digit):
10 9 8 7 6 5 4 3 2 1

PRINTED IN THE UNITED STATES OF AMERICA

PREFACE

In 1955, Sir Geroge Pickering, after having reviewed the data on morbidity and mortality in men and women with essential hypertension, concluded that "for any given level of arterial pressure, women fare better than men." Ever since then, it has remained a textbook opinion that hypertension is a less severe risk factor in the female than in the male population. As a consequence, women were very often treated with benign neglect, not only when they had hypertension but also when they suffered from other cardiovascular diseases.

As is outlined in *Hypertension in Postmenopausal Women*, a variety of recent studies have documented that, particularly after the menopause, the risk of hypertensive women suffering from heart attack, sudden cardiac death, stroke, and other cardiovascular morbidity and mortality is as high as or even exceeds that of hypertensive men. The menopause not only increases the prevalence of hypertension, but also exponentially accelerates the development of other cardiovascular risk factors such as insulin resistance, dyslipoproteinemia, and obesity. In concert, these cardiovascular risk factors exert a powerful impact on life expectancy in the postmenopausal female population. The present monograph serves to inform the practicing physician of the specific problems related to hypertension and other cardiovascular disorders in the menopause and to familiarize the reader with the epidemiology, pathophysiology, clinical findings, and therapeutic options in hypertensive women after the menopause. Although hormone replacement therapy has been shown to diminish the overall risk of cardiovascular morbidity and mortality, much remains to be learned about preventive aspects as well as the safety and efficacy of cardiovascular drug therapy in this special situation. It is hoped that *Hypertension in Postmenopausal Women* will be a practical and useful resource for helping the practicing physician to deal with this exceedingly common entity.

I would like to acknowledge the help of the Alton Ochsner Medical Foundation Medical Editing Department, under the direction of Marion Stafford, in the completion of this project. It has been a pleasure for me to work with Marcel Dekker, Inc., especially Sandra Beberman, Assistant Vice President, Medical Division.

Franz H. Messerli

CONTENTS

CONTRIBUTORS

Franz C. Aepfelbacher, M.D.   Department of Hypertension, Ochsner Clinic and Alton Ochsner Medical Foundation, New Orleans, Louisiana

Marcello Arca, M.D.   Staff Researcher, Istituto di Terapia Medica Sistematica, Università di Roma "La Sapienza," Rome, Italy

Gareth Beevers, M.D., F.R.C.P.   Professor of Medicine, University Department of Medicine, City Hospital, Birmingham, England

Paul E. Belchetz, M.A., M.D., M.Sc., F.R.C.P.   Consultant Physician/Endocrinologist, Department of Endocrinology, The General Infirmary at Leeds, Leeds, West Yorkshire, England

Leszek Bieniaszewski, M.D., Ph.D.   Postdoctoral Research Assistant, Hypertension and Cardiovascular Rehabilitation Unit, Department of Molecular and Cardiovascular Research, University of Leuven, Leuven, Belgium

Vera Bittner, M.D.   Associate Professor of Medicine, Division of Cardiovascular Disease, Department of Medicine, University of Alabama at Birmingham, Birmingham, Alabama

Karen D. Bradshaw, M.D.   Associate Professor, Department of Obstetrics and Gynecology, University of Texas Southwestern Medical Center, Dallas, Texas

Ivo Brosens, M.D., Ph.D.   Professor of Gynecology, Gynecology and Obstetrics Unit, Department of Developmental Biology, University of Leuven, Leuven, Belgium

Robert Fagard, M.D., Ph.D.   Professor of Medicine, Hypertension and Cardiovascular Rehabilitation Unit, Department of Molecular and Cardiovascular Research, University of Leuven, Leuven, Belgium

Thorsten Fischer, M.D.   Department II of Obstetrics and Gynecology, Hypertension Study Unit, University of Erlangen/ Nuernberg, Klinikum Nuernberg, Germany

Laura P. Fowlkes, M.D.   Division of Cardiovascular Diseases, University of Tennessee, Memphis, Memphis, Tennessee

Brenda Kramer-Coutinho, M.D.   Department of Obstetrics and Gynecology, University of Massachusetts Medical Center, Worcester, Massachusetts

Gregory Y. H. Lip, M.D., M.R.C.P.   Postdoctoral Research Fellow, University Department of Medicine, City Hospital, Birmingham, England

Douglas W. Losordo, M.D.   Assistant Professor of Medicine, Tufts University School of Medicine, and Division of Cardiovascular Medicine, St. Elizabeth's Medical Center, Boston, Massachusetts

Franz H. Messerli, M.D.   Department of Hypertension, Ochsner Clinic and Alton Ochsner Medical Foundation, New Orleans, Louisiana

Eric L. Michelson, M.D.   Professor, Division of Cardiovascular Diseases, Department of Medicine, Medical College of Pennsylvania and Hahnemann University, Philadelphia, Pennsylvania

Celia M. Oakley, M.D., F.R.C.P., F.A.C.C., F.E.S.C. Professor of Clinical Cardiology, The Royal Postgraduate Medical School, and Hammersmith Hospital, London, England

Suzanne Oparil, M.D. Professor of Medicine, Vascular Biology and Hypertension Program of the Division of Cardiovascular Disease, Department of Medicine, University of Alabama at Birmingham, Birmingham, Alabama

Veronica Ravnikar, M.D. Professor of Obstetrics and Gynecology and Director, Division of Reproductive Endocrinology, Department of Obstetrics and Gynecology, University of Massachusetts Medical Center, Worcester, Massachusetts

Roland E. Schmieder, M.D. Assistant Professor, Department of Clinical Nephrology, Hypertension Study Unit, University of Erlangen/Nuernberg, Klinikum Nuernberg, Nuernberg, Germany

Kelly Anne Spratt, D.O. Clinical Assistant Professor, Division of Cardiovascular Diseases, Medical College of Pennsylvania and Hahnemann University, Philadelphia, Pennsylvania

Jan A. Staessen, M.D., Ph.D. Lecturer, Hypertension and Cardiovascular Rehabilitation Unit, Department of Molecular and Cardiovascular Research, University of Leuven, Leuven, Belgium

Jay M. Sullivan, M.D. Chief, Division of Cardiovascular Diseases, University of Tennessee, Memphis, Memphis, Tennessee

J. D. Swales, M.A., M.D., F.R.C.P. Head, Department of Medicine and Therapeutics, University of Leicester and Leicester Royal Infirmary, Leicester, England

John Zarifis, M.D. Research Fellow, University Department of Medicine, City Hospital, Birmingham, England

1

Overview

Celia M. Oakley
The Royal Postgraduate Medical School
and Hammersmith Hospital
London, England

I. INTRODUCTION

Coronary heart disease is the leading cause of mortality in women (1). Although it has been regarded as a disease that mainly afflicts men, it accounts for about 250,000 deaths annually in women in the United States and 76,000 in the United Kingdom, figures that are only slightly less than those for men from this cause.

The cardiovascular health of women has received little attention (2–4). The focus of research, of campaigns to reduce cardiovascular disease, and of major trials of primary and secondary prevention of coronary artery disease have been either

1

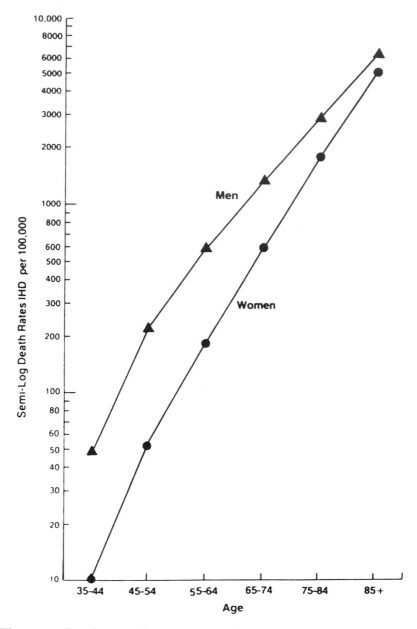

Figure 1 Death rates from ischemic heart disease among men and women aged 35 to 85+ years: United States, 1980 (rates per 100,000). (Data from the Natural Center for Health Statistics, U.S. Department of Health and Human Services.)

exclusively in males or with only minor recruitment of women, largely because of an upper-age cutoff and relatively few women in the age group studied (5).

Although cardiovascular deaths have been falling in the United States since the late 1960s and the past 10 years have seen the cardiac death rate fall by 25% in men in the United Kingdom, it has fallen by only 17% in women (6). While men in their fourth decade have five times the mortality of women from coronary heart disease, women start to catch up at an increasing rate after the menopause, reaching parity in old age (7,8) with men (Figure 1). The greater number of women compared with men living into old age with hypertension and coronary artery disease accounts for the closeness of the overall mortality figures.

II. RISK FACTORS AND CLINICAL FINDINGS

Most of the morbidity, disability, health care costs, and mortality occur in women after the menopause, but coronary artery disease, once almost nonexistent in younger women (except in severe familial hypercholesterolemia), is increasing and myocardial infarction is no longer uncommon. Younger women are smoking more, they are using oral contraceptives, and, believing that they are not at risk, they eat more saturated fats than men. They have also adopted an increasingly sedentary lifestyle from doing office jobs rather than housework. It has been suggested that coronary heart disease rates in younger women are moving closer to those in men because, as women adopt a lifestyle that is similar to men's, their advantage may be disappearing. In the 1950s twice as many men as women smoked. In the United Kingdom the figures are now similar. Death rates for British women are among the highest in the world—in Glasgow they are the highest (5).

Hypertension is a major risk factor for premature death and disability from stroke and heart failure, and it is the most frequent cause of end-stage renal failure. Hypertension is common in women, especially as they grow older, but since epidemiological studies have shown that women tolerate high blood pressure better, live longer, and have fewer complications than men with

similar blood pressure levels, raised blood pressure in women
has far too long been regarded as relatively benign.

A report published in London by the National Forum for
Coronary Heart Disease Prevention has called for a national
education campaign in the United Kingdom to increase awareness of the risks of heart disease in women (6).

Three large nationwide surveys carried out in the United
States between 1960 and 1980 showed that up to 22% of the total
population had a blood pressure equal to or greater than 160/95
mm Hg (9). The prevalence increased progressively with age and
was higher in blacks than in whites and in men than in women
except in older women. Younger black women have a higher
prevalence of hypertension than white women, catching up with
black men by the menopause, and have a higher cardiovascular
mortality in their younger years than white women.

It is now well recognized that left ventricular hypertrophy is
not a benign adaptive response to hypertension but a major risk
factor for sudden death and heart failure. A complex interplay of
many genetic factors (most still to be worked out) contribute not
only to the development of hypertension but also to hypertrophy.
This occurs not only in the myocardium but also in the smooth
muscle of the systemic resistance vessels. Polymorphisms of the
angiotensin converting enzyme (ACE) gene may contribute to
the risk of myocardial infarction as well as to a fatal outcome
from it (10). Clustering of risk factors for cardiovascular disease
determines that hypertensives also have a higher prevalence of
insulin resistance, non-insulin-dependent diabetes, hyperlipidemia, and abdominal obesity—a metabolic syndrome that is
important in women as well as in men (11).

The increase in prevalence of coronary heart disease after
the menopause—previously thought to be only an effect of
aging—is also attributable to loss of estrogens, with associated
adverse changes both in lipid levels and in vascular resistance.
Data from the Framingham heart study showed that total cholesterol levels in women are lower than those in men up to the age of
about 50, but that, while male cholesterol levels subsequently
remain about the same, cholesterol levels in women start to rise
from the age of about 40, exceeding those in men by the age of 50

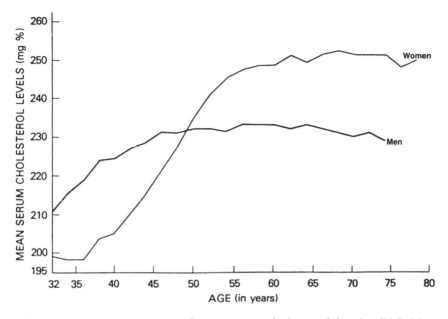

Figure 2 Average age trends in serum cholesterol levels. (U.S. National Data from the Framingham Study.)

and thereafter (7) (Figure 2). Low-density-lipoprotein levels rise after the menopause, with little change in total high-density lipoprotein (except for a fall in major protective HDL-2 component of cholesterol). Thus, the favorable ratio of high- to low-density lipoprotein present in younger women deteriorates after the menopause, as it does in women who have undergone oophorectomy or premature menopause, both of which are well known to increase the risk of coronary heart disease. Recent studies have shown evidence of estrogen receptors in the smooth muscle of coronary arteries whose expression was most evident in premenopausal subjects without coronary artery disease (12). Hormone replacement therapy changes the lipid profile back to resemble that seen before the menopause, lowers blood pressure, is antithrombotic, and reduces the incidence of myocardial infarction. Administration of estradiol-17-β may even be a useful adjunct in the treatment of angina in postmenopausal women with coronary disease, possibly through a coronary vasodilator and calcium antagonist effect (13).

Loss of estrogens may also contribute to a rise in blood pressure and to the increase in cardiovascular events, stroke, and myocardial infarction after the menopause. In contrast, synthetic estrogens given in nonphysiological dosage for oral contraception increase cardiovascular risk by elevating triglycerides, blood pressure, and plasma insulin and raising the hemostatic profile through an increase in coagulation factors. The synthetic progestogens are androgenic and may compound the risk. The adverse effects of oral contraceptives containing synthetic estrogens and progestogens may be enhanced and the risks increased in women over the age of 35, particularly if they smoke and are overweight. The fact that it takes more than 20 years for the fatality rate from coronary heart disease in women to reach that of men of the same age may be because of the slow natural history of atherogenesis, but oral contraceptive use—often for more than 20 years—may be contributing to the trend for women's cardiovascular mortality figures to be catching up with men's.

In the past, medical interest has focused on the reasons for the differential risks of cardiovascular disease between men and women rather than on attempting to reduce the prevalence of such disease in women. The big primary prevention trials, which excluded women, have resulted in a shortage of information on risk factors in women and on mortality differences between women from different nations and different cultural and ethnic groups (14). We know that a Spanish or Japanese woman of 70 can look forward to the probability of living until almost 90 whereas a Scottish woman of the same age may not anticipate reaching even 80.

III. DIAGNOSIS AND TREATMENT OF CORONARY HEART DISEASE

Important gender differences exist in the clinical presentation of coronary heart disease but account only in part for major differences in diagnosis, treatment, and prognosis (15–17). Anginal pain is the usual initial presentation of coronary heart disease in women, and an early Framingham study showed the prognosis of angina to be more favorable in women than in men, with 25% of men with angina having an infarct within 5 years compared with only half that number of women (18). The reason for this seemingly better prognosis is an increased prevalence of chest pain although the epicardial coronary arteries appear to be normal. As is well known, this syndrome X has a good prognosis, but it is surprising that controversy still rages concerning whether the chest pain is based on myocardial ischemia (so-called microvascular angina). The prognosis of angina in women with disease of the epicardial coronary arteries may therefore be no better, or even worse, than in men.

While the threshold to somatic pain may be lower in the sufferers of syndrome X than in other subjects, the threshold in women to the perception of the pain of myocardial infarction appears to be higher than in men. Their greater age, a high prevalence of diabetes, and high tolerance to or atypical nature of the pain may all contribute to the late presentation of women with coronary artery disease, with myocardial infarction and probably also angina. Because they are older at presentation, more of the women also have multivessel coronary disease when first seen (15–17). Cardiac symptoms in females are often overlooked by both the patients and their doctors, with the result that women with myocardial infarction have longer delay before admission to hospital, get less intensive treatment, receive less secondary preventive therapy, and have poorer residual left ventricular function and a worse survival chance than men. Of 800 patients admitted to the coronary care unit of the London Chest Hospital over the 5-year period from 1988 to 1992, one in three women died within 6 months compared to one in six men. The women were older, but their excess risk persisted after adjustment for age, other baseline variables, and indices of severity of infarction. The women tended to be treated less often with thrombolytic agents, and substantially fewer women than men were discharged taking beta-blockers (15). A study in Nottingham during 1989 and 1990 showed that women with myocardial infarction took longer than men to arrive at the hospital. They were less likely to be admitted to the coronary care unit and were therefore also less likely to receive thrombolytic treatment. They seemed to have more severe infarcts with higher Killip classes and thus a slightly higher mortality during admission; in addition, they were found to be less likely than men to receive secondary prophylaxis with beta-blockers or aspirin (16).

The exercise ECG is well known to be less accurate for the diagnosis of ischemic heart disease in women than in men, and exercise echocardiography may be more specific than ST-segment analysis for the diagnosis of coronary artery disease in women with a high pretest probability of having coronary artery disease. Echocardiography may also have greater prognostic significance than the exercise ECG (20).

Although women have a higher mortality rate after myocardial infarction than men, they are less frequently referred for cardiac catheterization (21) and therefore have less chance to benefit from coronary angioplasty or coronary artery bypass graft surgery. This seems to be because of lower pretest prediction of coronary disease by their physicians (21) and possibly also because of expectation of a worse outcome—although the procedural outcome of coronary angioplasty for post–myocardial infarction ischemia is similar in women and men, so concerns over the safety of coronary angioplasty in women should not adversely influence decisions (22). On the other hand, an increased operative mortality in women after coronary bypass surgery is probably explained by their more advanced age, more advanced coronary artery disease at referral, smaller coronary arteries, and more diabetes and hypertension with more left ventricular hypertrophy and poorer myocardial function (19). Nevertheless, the survivors of coronary surgery show excellent long-term benefit comparable with that in men (23).

Coronary heart disease in the elderly is a problem affecting more women than men, and coronary heart disease in women has been calculated to cost the United States Health Care Service more than coronary heart disease in men (5). Gender bias against aggressive intervention and treatment may have been aggravated by atypical clinical syndromes.

The allegation that doctors underinvestigate and undertreat women with coronary heart disease has been countered by claims (in the United Kingdom) that (in the United States) the level of revascularization in women is more appropriate than it is in men (5). This may well be half true, U.K. perception being that the rate of revascularization in American men is excessive!

Whatever the gender differences in atherogenesis, chest pain, and prevalence and mortality of myocardial infarction, there is no justification for treating men and women differently after coronary heart disease has been diagnosed. Women with coronary heart disease do not do well, and better methods of prevention and early identification are needed. This particular problem has been largely ignored (24).

REFERENCES

1. Wenger NK, Speroff L, Packard B. Cardiovascular health and disease in women. N Engl J Med 1993; 329:247–256.
2. Manolio TA, Harlan WR. Research on coronary disease in women: political or scientific imperative? Br Heart J 1993; 69:1–2.
3. The Yentl Syndrome. N Engl J Med 1991; 325:274–276.
4. Khaw KT. Where are the women in studies of coronary heart disease? Br Med J 1993; 306:1145–1146.
5. Findlay IN, Cunningham D, Dargie HJ. The rights of women (editorial). Br Heart J 1994; 71(5):401–403.
6. Report from the National Forum for Coronary Heart Disease Prevention. Are Women Special? London, 1994.
7. Kannel WB, Hjortland MC, McNamara PM, Gordon T. Menopause and the risk of cardiovascular disease: The Framingham Study. Ann Intern Med 1976; 85:447–452.
8. Colditz GA, Willett WC, Stampfer MJ, Rosner B, Speizer FE, Hennekens CH. Menopause and the risk of coronary heart disease in women. N Engl J Med 1987; 316:1105–1110.
9. Stellman JM, ed. Women's occupational health: Medical, social and legal implications. Prev Med 1978; 7:281.
10. Evans AE, Poirier O, Kee F, Lecerf L, McCrum E, Falconer T, Crane

J, O'Rourke DF, Cambien F. Polymorphisms of the angiotensin-converting enzyme gene in subjects who die from coronary heart disease. Quart J Med 1994; 87(4):211–214.

11. Hauner H, Bognar E, Blum A. Body fat distribution and its association with metabolic and hormonal risk factors in women with angiographically assessed coronary artery disease: Evidence for the presence of a metabolic syndrome. Atherosclerosis 1994; 105 (2):209–216.

12. Losordo DW, Kearney M, Kim EA, Kejanowski J, Isner JM. Variable expression of the estrogen receptor in normal and atherosclerotic coronary arteries of premenopausal women. Circulation 1994; 89(4):1501–1510.

13. Rosano GM, Sarrel PM, Poole-Wilson PA, Collins P. Beneficial effect of oestrogen on exercise-induced myocardial ischaemia in women with coronary artery disease. Lancet 1993; 342:133–136.

14. Kitler ME. Coronary disease: are there gender differences? Eur Heart J 1994; 15(3):409–417.

15. Wilkinson P, Laji K, Ranjadayalan K, Parsons L, Timmis AD. Acute myocardial infarction in women: survival analysis in first six months. Br Med J 1994; 309:566–569.

16. Clarke KW, Gray D, Keating NA, Hampton JR. Do women with acute myocardial infarction receive the same treatment as men? Br Med J 1994; 309:563–566.

17. Becker RC, Terrin M, Ross R, Knatterud GL, Desvigne-Nickens P, Gore JM, Braunwald E. The Thrombolysis in Myocardial Infarction Investigators. Comparison of clinical outcomes for women and men after acute myocardial infarction. Ann Intern Med 1994; 120(8):638–645.

18. Kannel WB, Feinleib M. Natural history of angina pectoris in the Framingham Study: prognosis and survival. Am J Cardiol 1972; 29:154.

19. Iwasaka T, Sugiura T, Abe Y, Karakawa M, Matsui Y, Wakayama Y, Negahama Y, Tamura K, Inada M. Residual left ventricular pump function following acute myocardial infarction in postmenopausal diabetic women. Coronary Artery Dis 1994; 5(3):237–242.

20. Williams MJ, Marwick TH, O'Gorman D, Foale RA. Comparison of exercise echocardiography with an exercise score to diagnose coronary artery disease in women. Am J Cardiol 1994; 74:435–438.

21. Mark DB, Shaw LK, DeLong ER, Califf RM, Pryor DB. Absence of sex bias in the referral of patients for cardiac catheterization. N Engl J Med 1994; 330(16):1101–1106.

22. Welty FK, Mittleman MA, Healy RW, Muller JE, Shubrooks SJ Jr. Similar results of percutaneous transluminal coronary angioplasty for women and men with postmyocardial infarction ischemia. J Am Coll Cardiol 1994; 23(1):35–39.

23. Rahimtoola SH, Bennett AJ, Grunkemeier GL, Block P, Starr A. Survival at 15 to 18 years after coronary bypass surgery for angina in women. Circulation 1993; 88:II71–II78.

24. Kuhn FE, Rackley CE. Coronary artery disease in women: Risk factors, evaluation, treatment and prevention. Arch Intern Med 1993; 153(23):2626–2636.

2

Estrogen Receptors and Cardiovascular Disease

Douglas W. Losordo

Tufts University School of Medicine
and St. Elizabeth's Medical Center
Boston, Massachusetts

I. EPIDEMIOLOGICAL EVIDENCE OF ATHEROPROTECTIVE EFFECTS OF ESTROGEN

The relative protection from coronary atherosclerosis conferred upon premenopausal women is well established. Heberden (quoted in Ref. 1) commented on the sex difference in the incidence of angina pectoris in 1803. Others have documented the lower incidence of coronary atherosclerosis in premenopausal females in epidemiological and autopsy studies (2–6). The increased incidence of atherosclerosis in women who undergo premature menopause has also been well described (7–12). Finally, there is increasing evidence that treatment with replacement estrogen (E_2) after menopause will reduce cardiovascular mortality (13–15), although the role of progesterone continues to be debated (15,16).

II. EXPERIMENTAL ANIMAL EVIDENCE DEMONSTRATING CHANGES IN ARTERIAL MORPHOLOGY DUE TO ESTROGEN ADMINISTRATION OR DEPRIVATION

Animal studies have provided further evidence of estrogen's effects on the vascular system. Estrogen treatment prevented collagen and elastin accumulation in the aortic wall in normotensive rats (17) and thickening of the aorta in hypertensive rats (18), and similarly suppressed atherosclerosis in primate coronary arteries (19). Alternatively, progesterone (Pr) administered alone resulted in an increase in fatty-streak formation in castrated baboons, whereas animals receiving E_2 and Pr together had the fewest lesions (20). Thus, in an intact animal preparation, multiple studies have suggested an effect of sex steroids on vascular biology, specifically alluding to an antiproliferative effect of estrogen and raising the question of a synergistic effect of progesterone. These studies lend experimental support to the hypothesis brought forward by epidemiological studies that female sex hormones are protective against coronary atherosclerosis. What these studies do not address, however, is the mechanism(s) by which the presence of estrogen is translated into an effect on the biology of the arterial wall.

III. ESTROGEN'S ATHEROPROTECTIVE EFFECT IS PARTIALLY EXPLAINED BY ALTERATION IN SERUM LIPIDS

Endogenous and exogenous estrogens have been observed to alter the levels of serum lipids (8,13,16) and lipid metabolism in humans (21,22). In experimental animals fed an atherogenic diet, administration of estrogen inhibited (23–25) or reversed (26) atheroma formation, associated with reversion of lipid levels toward normal. Thus, well-established experimental animal data has demonstrated an atheroprotective effect of estrogen. These studies also demonstrate that estrogen administration results in a more normal lipid profile in animals fed a high-cholesterol diet. Furthermore, these studies are corroborated by human evidence demonstrating a favorable alteration in lipid levels in the presence of endogenous or exogenously administered estrogen, as well as changes in lipid metabolism that would explain these alterations in lipoprotein profiles.

IV. THE ROLE OF PROGESTERONE IN MODIFYING THE ESTROGEN EFFECT ON SERUM LIPIDS

Early human clinical data suggested that progesterone tended to mitigate the beneficial effect of estrogen on serum lipids (16,22). More recent studies, however, have demonstrated no significant attenuation of the salutary effects on serum lipid profiles induced by estrogen replacement in postmenopausal women (15,27).

The experimental animal and human data provide a partial explanation for the salutary effect of estrogen on the incidence of coronary atherosclerosis. The changes in serum lipids noted in human patients, however, fail to fully account for the discrepancy in the incidence of coronary disease between men and premenopausal women (14,28).

V. EXPERIMENTAL ANIMAL DATA DEMONSTRATING CHANGE IN ARTERIAL VASOMOTION SUGGEST DIRECT ESTROGEN EFFECT ON ARTERIAL WALL

A direct effect of estrogen on the arterial wall is suggested by animal and human experimental data. Vasodilation in response to estrogen administration was first noted in the rabbit ear artery (29) and later in human umbilical (30) and primate coronary arteries (31). Gender differences in the contractile response of the aorta in rats have been shown (32), as has estrogen-dependent sexual dimorphism of rat vascular smooth-muscle cells (VSMCs). Recently, acute administration of estradiol has been shown to attenuate abnormal coronary vasomotor responses in postmenopausal women (33,34). While this experimental evidence furthers the suggestion of a direct estrogen effect on vascular tissue, neither a systemic effect nor a non-receptor-mediated effect of estrogen is excluded by these studies.

VI. ISOLATED VASCULAR SMOOTH-MUSCLE CELLS RESPOND TO ESTROGEN

Examination of VSMCs in culture, however, has provided further data suggesting a direct estrogen effect on vascular tissue. Nichols et al. (35) demonstrated decreased protein synthesis in rat VSMCs in culture when they are exposed to estrogen. Isolating vascular tissue from the systemic effects of sex steroid administration in this study, therefore, provided evidence of a *direct* effect of E_2 on cells of the artery wall.

VII. IDENTIFICATION OF ESTROGEN RECEPTOR IN VASCULAR TISSUE

Estrogen, like all steroids, acts by binding to a specific receptor. Establishing a direct, genomically mediated mechanism of E_2 action on the vessel wall therefore requires demonstration of estrogen receptor (ER) in the target tissue. ER has been demonstrated in canine peripheral (36) and coronary (37) arteries, in cultured rat aortic VSMCs (38), and in human vascular endothelial cells (39). Smooth-muscle cells at low passage in culture have been shown to retain the ER expression of the parent tissue (40). Finally, an association between E_2 stimulation (in these ER-containing tissues) and physiological effect has been demonstrated (37,41,42). The actual function of the ER, however, and the cellular mechanisms that translate E_2–ER interaction into physiological effect on the arterial wall remain to be defined.

VIII. CELL BIOLOGY OF THE ESTROGEN RECEPTOR

The ER belongs to the nuclear receptor superfamily, a class of ligand-activated transcription factors that includes 30 receptors including steroid hormone and thyroid hormone receptors, as well as vitamin D3 and retinoic acid receptors. Classic steroid hormone receptors form homodimers and recognize short palindromic DNA sequences (steroid response elements) often located upstream from their target genes (43–45). Recent evidence, however, has challenged the assumption that all nuclear receptors act via a single unique palindromic DNA sequence (46).

Early studies suggested that the unbound ER is located in the cytoplasm and that after binding its ligand the receptor translocates to the nucleus due to an increase in the receptor's affinity for chromatin (47). More recent work, however, has demonstrated both occupied and unoccupied ER residing in the nucleus (48,49). ER probably interacts with DNA, chromosomal proteins, and a nuclear chromatin scaffolding structure that may regulate translation and transcriptional activity (50–53).

Clones of the 2.2 kb ER cDNA have been sequenced from the human breast cancer cell line MCF-7 demonstrating an open reading frame of 1785 nucleotides sufficient to encode ER (54). The mRNA codes for a 66 kDa protein with strong structural homology to glucocorticoid receptor as well as to the v-erb-A protein of the oncogenic avian erythroblastosis virus. Conservation of the cysteine-rich and hydrophobic regions in these sequences supports the assertion that they are important functional domains, although the complete significance of this homology has not been clarified.

IX. MECHANISMS OF ESTROGENIC CONTROL OF PROLIFERATION

Much of what has been learned regarding the biological and biochemical effects of the E_2–ER interaction has been derived from study of human breast cancer cells. In these in vitro model systems, E_2 induces a number of enzymes involved in nucleic acid synthesis (55,56). DNA synthesis by scavenger and de novo pathways is also stimulated (57). E_2 regulates thymidine kinase and dihydrofolate at the mRNA and translational levels, although the genes that are regulated in this process have not been identified (56,58,59).

In fact, the exact mechanisms of regulation of cell proliferation by E_2 remain to be clarified. Several hypotheses have been explored regarding the E_2-proliferation link that are useful to consider as a framework for examining the E_2–ER role in arterial-wall biology. All these putative mechanisms have been developed in an attempt to understand the role of estrogen as a synergist or catalyst of proliferative activity, a role directly opposite of that envisioned for E_2 in atherosclerosis. Still, it is helpful to consider these same types of actions, if acting in reverse, as theoretical possibilities for E_2 action on hVSMC biology. A *direct positive* mechanism would have E_2 directly triggering the proliferation of target cells. A direct mitogenic effect of E_2 has been shown, for example, in the prepubertal rat uterus (60). In an *indirect-positive* model, E_2 induces the production of growth factors, which then results in target cell division (61). In this model the growth factors are produced by cells other than the target cells, while in an *autocrine* mechanism the target cells themselves elucidate the second messenger (62).

Recently estrogens have been shown to mediate growth arrest and differentiation in a neuroblastoma cell line (63). This study demonstrated the involvement of activated ER in metabolic changes leading cells toward a differentiated/nonproliferating state.

X. THE ROLE OF PROGESTERONE IN MODIFYING ESTROGEN–ESTROGEN RECEPTOR BIOLOGY

Many eukaryotic genes are under the control of multiple hormones, and steroid-response elements can be found in multiple copies or tightly clustered with other *cis*-acting DNA elements (64). Synergism between the estrogen receptor and the progesterone receptor has been demonstrated in vitro, but this effect does not appear to result from cooperative binding to their respective response elements (64). In addition, certain progestins can exhibit estrogenic potential; this effect does appear to be mediated by the ER, as evidenced by its inhibition by antiestrogens (65). Important E_2–Pr interactions have been reported by several investigators (66–70). The exact nature of this interaction remains to be well characterized.

The findings of prior investigations of the effect of the E_2–ER interaction on arterial biology can be summarized as follows:

1. Epidemiological evidence suggests a protective role of estrogen against coronary atherosclerosis.
2. While it is clear that the presence of estrogen has a salutary effect on serum lipid levels, the atheroprotective effect of estrogen cannot be *entirely* explained by the changes in serum lipids.
3. Experimental animal evidence has demonstrated decreased proliferative activity of cells of the arterial wall, when they are stimulated by injury, hypertension, or atherogenic diets, when estrogen is administered.
4. Estrogen has been shown to change the behavior of isolated vascular tissue derived from experimental animals.
5. ER expression has been documented in the vascular tissues of some animals and in endothelial cells of humans.

Thus, epidemiological and experimental evidence points to a significant effect of estrogen on vascular biology and suggests the possibility of a direct estrogen effect on cells of the arterial wall.

Based on this previous experimental data, our laboratory embarked on a series of preliminary investigations to determine if a direct action of estrogen on human vascular tissue was a plausible explanation for the apparent atheroprotective effect of estrogen in human patients.

While part of the atheroprotective effect of E_2 is mediated by amelioration of serum lipid patterns, a portion of E_2's beneficial effect is not explained by changes in lipids. We theorized that a direct effect of E_2 on the arterial wall was also possible. To exert a direct genomic effect, however, expression of a functional ER would be required. Accordingly, we performed a series of investigations to identify such a receptor in hVSMCs (71).

A. Verification and Precise Quantification of ER Expression in hVSMCs

Cultures of hVSMCs were grown by the explant outgrowth technique as previously reported. This technique has been used successfully in our laboratory to derive cultures of hVSMCs from normal arteries as well as from atherosclerotic plaque obtained by directional atherectomy (72). The identity of the cells in culture is confirmed by staining with antibody to smooth-muscle α-actin.

Assay for ER in this system was performed by adapting a technique previously established for receptor assay in breast carcinoma tissue to the assay of ER in hVSMC culture (38,73). Characteristic saturation plots were generated from these studies (71). The binding of receptors was saturable in the concentration range studied, similar to results obtained with ER binding in VSMC culture of other species (38). The binding curve indicates specific binding of the radiolabeled ligand to ER in hVSMC. The binding could not be caused by nonspecific interaction of labeled steroid, as this is controlled for by the series of experiments performed in the presence of 200-fold excess unlabeled DES. From these same data the precise quantity of estrogen receptors is calculated to equal 1.16×10^{-13} M/10^6 hVSMCs. These data also represent a high-affinity estrogen receptor as is indicated by the calculated Kd of 8×10^{-9}.

These data represent the first verification of high-affinity ERs in hVSMCs, and they have since been confirmed by others (74).

B. Estradiol-Dependent Binding of hVSMC ER to an Estrogen-Responsive Element in Vitro

Steroid-responsive elements are inducible regulatory DNA sequences that interact with their receptors and modulate transcription of target genes. The "estrogen responsive element" (ERE) has been shown to bind the ER only when the latter is induced by its ligand. Previous studies have demonstrated a 13 bp palindrome (5'–GGTCACAGTGACC–3') that is the minimal DNA sequence sufficient for significant estrogen induction and specific binding of ER (75,76). The interaction of hormone-bound ER with the ERE has been shown to alter the transcriptional efficiency of ERE-containing genes. Efficient binding of ligand-induced ER to the ERE is therefore a useful measure of the functional integrity of putative receptors.

We examined the ability of ERs from hVSMCs to bind ERE using gel-mobility assays. This assay is based on the fact that protein-bound DNA migrates more slowly through a polyacrylamide gel than unbound DNA. In the presence of estrogen, the ER should form a complex with the ERE. By labeling the response element with ^{32}P, the complexes can be identified by their altered electrophoretic mobility.

In these studies, specific and ligand-dependent binding of hVSMC ER to its cognate response element is demonstrated (71). Only the combination of extract from E_2-exposed cells and labeled ERE probe produces the "shifted" band corresponding to the DNA–receptor complex.

Confirmation of the presence and functional integrity of ER in hVSMCs suggests that a *direct* effect of E_2 on human arteries is a possibility. If the atheroprotective effect of estrogen is mediated, in part, by *direct* action on the arterial wall, it is possible that the occurrence of coronary atherosclerosis in female patients may be precipitated by one of two events: 1) the loss of circulating *ligand* (estrogen) or 2) absolute or relative lack of (estrogen) *receptor* expression by target cells in the arterial wall. The first of these two situations occurs when patients reach menopause, and this is associated with an increase in the incidence of coronary disease. The latter possibility, however, has not previously been investigated.

C. Demonstration of Decreased ER Expression in Atherosclerotic Coronary Arteries

Accordingly, an investigation was performed to test the hypothesis that premature atherosclerosis in female patients may be mediated by a failure of target cells in the vessel wall to adequately express ER, therefore abrogating the possibility of atheroprotection by circulating estrogen. We surveyed the autopsy records of St. Elizabeth's Hospital for the past 10 years to identify pre- and postmenopausal patients with normal and atherosclerotic coronary arteries. Our intention was to identify as many premenopausal subjects as possible, since the testing of our hypothesis would be based largely on our examination of these tissues. The distribution of subjects identified in our search of the records is shown in Table 1; they included 18 premenopausal and 22 postmenopausal women. The coronary arteries of these pa-

Table 1　Distribution and Ages of Patients According to Menopausal Status at Time of Death and the Presence or Absence of Coronary Atherosclerosis

	n	Age (mean ± SEM)
Premenopausal	18	31.6 ± 1.9
Normal	12	31.2 ± 2.1[a]
Atherosclerotic	6	32.6 ± 4.3[a]
Postmenopausal	22	71.8 ± 2.3
Normal	9	75.1 ± 5.0[a]
Atherosclerotic	13	69.4 ± 1.7[a]

p = NS.
Source: Ref 71. Reprinted with permission. Copyright 1994 American Heart Association.

tients were classified as normal in 21 subjects and atherosclerotic in 19 subjects, based on the histological examination of the specimens.

Evaluation of ER expression in these coronary artery specimens was performed using a monoclonal antibody to the ER (H222spγ, Abbott Labs, Abbott Park, IL). While this technique was designed for use on fresh tissue, modifications in the preparations of specimens have permitted detection of ER in formalin-fixed, paraffin-embedded tissue (77). To ensure the reliability of this technique, positive control tissue consisting of a breast carcinoma, previously shown by radioligand-binding assays to express high levels of ER, was used in all the immunohistochemical staining runs on the coronary specimens. Examples of coronary artery specimens from premenopausal women with normal and atherosclerotic arteries are shown in Figures 1 and 2, respectively.

ER expression in the coronary arteries of all subjects studied is shown in Table 2. Of 21 normal arteries studied, 15 showed evidence of ER expression, while of 19 atherosclerotic arteries, 13 showed no evidence of ER expression when assayed immunohistochemically. Contingency table analysis revealed that the differences between these groups were statistically significant, with $p = 0.0117$.

Interestingly, when the results of the immunohistochemical staining for ER expression in the coronary arteries of postmenopausal subjects were analyzed separately (Table 2, right), the impact of ER expression was no longer evident. Of nine normal coronary arteries of postmenopausal patients, ER expression was evident in five and absent in four. Only four of 12 atherosclerotic arteries showed evidence of ER expression. The differences in ER expression between these groups did not achieve statistical significance.

When the results of ER staining of coronary arteries of premenopausal women were analyzed separately, however, the association between ER expression and absence of coronary atherosclerosis was again evident, and apparently was responsible for the statistical association noted in the total population studied. Of 12 normal arteries, ER expression was shown immunohisto-

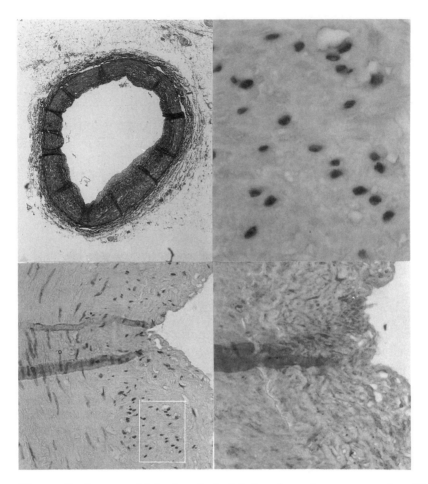

Figure 1 Immunohistochemical staining for estrogen receptor. (Top left) elastic-trichrome stain reveals minimal intimal thickening in this coronary artery specimen from a premenopausal female who died from noncardiac causes. (Bottom left) low-power (100×) view of the same artery after staining with monoclonal antibody to estrogen receptor. Blue staining of cell nuclei indicates positive staining for estrogen receptor. Artifact is due to folding of specimen during processing for histology. Area enclosed in white border is shown at high power above right. (Top right) high-power (330×) view of same section of premenopausal coronary artery demonstrating immunological evidence of estrogen

chemically in 10, while five of six atherosclerotic arteries showed no evidence of ER expression. The differences were highly statistically significant ($p = 0.0062$).

These results demonstrate a strong association between ER expression and the absence of coronary atherosclerosis in premenopausal women. The absence of this relationship in postmenopausal women could be explained by the estrogen-deficient state of the subjects, making the presence of the receptor alone insufficient to exert an atheroprotective effect. These data provide further evidence suggesting a *direct* action of estrogen in protecting arteries from atherosclerosis. Still, the mere association between ER expression and the absence of coronary atherosclerosis in premenopausal women does not establish a cause-and-effect relationship, nor does it provide any information regarding the functionality of the receptor.

D. Immunocytochemical Staining for ER in Cultured hVSMCs

To confirm the presence of ER protein in cultured hVSMCs, a second antibody to human ER was used for immunostaining (Figure 3). This antibody, designated ER-21 (generously provided by Geoffrey Greene, University of Chicago), is a rabbit polyclonal antibody directed at the N-terminus of the ER.

E. Antiproliferative Effect of Estrogen on hVSMCs

Having 1) established ER expression in hVSMCs, 2) determined that ERs derived from hVSMCs are functionally intact, and

---

receptor, indicated by intense blue-black staining of nuclei. (Bottom right) adjacent section of same artery stained with antibody to smooth-muscle α-actin to confirm presence of vascular smooth muscle cells in the region of the artery also positive for estrogen receptor expression. (From Ref. 71. Reprinted with permission. Copyright 1994 American Heart Association.)

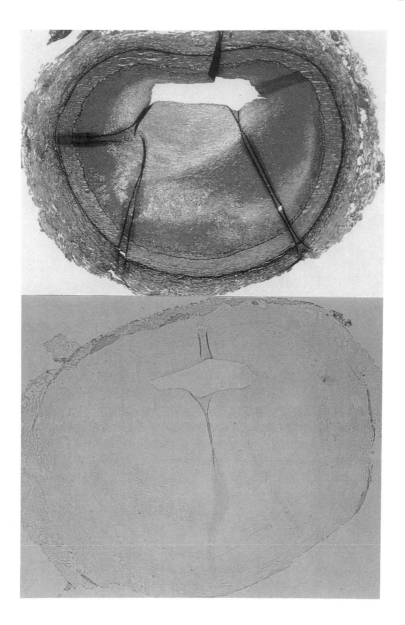

3) demonstrated a relationship between ER expression and the absence of atherosclerosis in human arteries, our next goal was to provide further evidence of transcriptional regulation of these receptors. The goal of the next series of preliminary experiments, therefore, was to observe hVSMCs in culture for different patterns of behavior in response to varying concentrations of estrogen in the cell-culture medium. In this series of experiments we evaluated the effect of estrogen on proliferative activity as determined by thymidine incorporation.

In hVSMC cultures the cells that were grown in medium supplemented by male serum demonstrated significantly greater thymidine incorporation than those cells from the same population grown in medium supplemented by serum from female patients. Furthermore, the proliferative effect of male serum on hVSMCs in culture was mitigated in part by the addition of estradiol to the culture medium.

The effect of estradiol on proliferative activity of hVSMCs in culture is further supported by a dose-response relationship, with higher doses of estradiol resulting in incremental inhibition of proliferative activity. Cultures of hVSMCs derived from the same artery were grown under identical conditions in defined media until serum with varying concentrations of estradiol was added. Tritiated thymidine was added to the culture medium, and thymidine incorporation was assayed after 48 hours. Male serum, with the lowest estradiol concentration, induced the greatest proliferative activity of cultured hVSMCs. With the addition of 10^{-9} M estradiol, the proliferative activity of the cells was significantly diminished. A further decrease in proliferative ac-

---

Figure 2 Immunohistochemical staining for estrogen receptor. (Top) elastic-trichrome stain of severely atherosclerotic artery from a premenopausal woman reveals extensive disease. (Bottom) photomicrograph (100×) of same coronary artery stained with antibody for estrogen receptor demonstrates no evidence of estrogen receptor protein. (From Ref. 71. Reprinted with permission. Copyright 1994 American Heart Association.)

Table 2 Results of Immunostaining for Estrogen Receptor in
Coronary Arteries: Distribution of Coronary Arteries Examined
According to Presence or Absence of Atherosclerosis and
Immunohistological Evidence of Estrogen Receptor

Estrogen receptor	All patients[a]		Premenopausal[b]		Postmenopausal[c]	
	Normal	Athero-sclerotic	Normal	Athero-sclerotic	Normal	Athero-sclerotic
+	15	6	10	1	5	4
−	6	13	2	5	4	8

[a]$p = 0.0117$.
[b]$p = 0.0062$.
[c]p = not significant
Source: Ref. 71. Reprinted with permission. Copyright 1994 American Heart Association.

tivity was demonstrated when the estradiol concentration was
increased further to 10^{-7} M.

F. Evidence of a Receptor-Mediated Effect of Estrogen on hVSMC Proliferation

Tamoxifen is widely known as an "antiestrogen" for its role in
treating estrogen-sensitive breast carcinoma. Tamoxifen does
bind to the ER and will inhibit the effects of estrogen, when it is
present in significant concentrations, in tissues that express a
functional ER. Tamoxifen is also, however, a partial antagonist in
its own right that will mimic, to some extent, the effects of estrogen on ER-positive tissue. In fact, recent clinical data suggest that
tamoxifen may be atheroprotective in postmenopausal women (78).

To examine the question of whether the antiproliferative
effect of E_2 on hVSMCs is mediated by a ligand–receptor interaction, studies were performed examining the effect of the pure
ER antagonist ICI 182780 (generously supplied by Zeneca Pharmaceuticals) to determine whether the antiproliferative effect of
E_2 on hVSMCs is mediated by ER.

In studies using human serum or dextran charcoal stripped

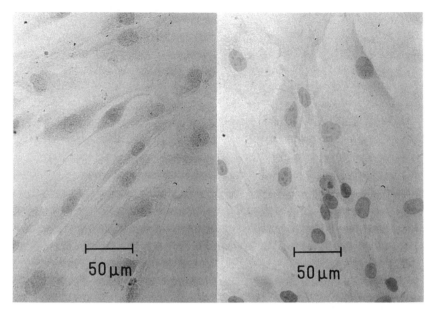

Figure 3 Immunocytochemical staining, estrogen receptor. Human vascular smooth muscle cells in culture stained with antibody (ER-21) to human estrogen receptor. (Left) positively stained cells contrast with (right) negative controls which show only evidence of hematoxylin counterstain. (100×). (From Ref. 71. Reprinted with permission. Copyright 1994 American Heart Association.)

FBS, the pure ERA mitigated the antiproliferative effect of E_2 when it was added to the culture medium before the E_2-containing culture medium.

G. Progesterone Does Not Diminish the Antiproliferative Effect of E_2 on hVSMCs

The same experimental design was used to examine the effect of the presence of progesterone (Pr) on the antiproliferative effect of E_2 on hVSMCs. In these studies, Pr (10^{-7} and 10^{-5} M) was added to the culture medium alone and in combination with E_2, and thymidine incorporation was again evaluated. The addition of E_2

was again shown to inhibit proliferation of hVSMCs. These assays also show that the antiproliferative effect of E_2 was not altered by the addition of Pr. Thus, Pr does not negate or enhance the apparent antiproliferative effect of E_2 on hVSMCs in culture.

These preliminary investigations, therefore, suggest that the presence of progesterone does not alter the direct effect of E_2 on hVSMC proliferative activity. The precise nature of the interaction between E_2 and Pr as it relates to hVSMC biology remains to be elucidated, however.

H. Proliferative Activity of Individual hVSMCs Is Inversely Related to ER Expression

Further evidence of a functional role of the ER in hVSMC biology is provided by the observation that individual hVSMCs expressing high levels of ER show diminished proliferative activity while cells with low levels of ER expression show evidence of entering the cell cycle.

Double-labeling studies were performed utilizing autoradiographic detection of ER expression in individual cells combined with immunohistochemical detection of bromodeoxyuridine incorporation as an index of proliferative activity. The purpose here was twofold. First, the autoradiographic technique would permit detection of ER expression among individual cells within the culture population. Previous evaluations of human breast cancer cell culture populations have indicated that only a percentage of cells, even in a population of cells known to express high levels of ER, are expressing ER at significant levels. Second, as noted above, it would provide the opportunity to study any relationship between ER expression and proliferative activity within individual cells. Figure 4 shows an example of the application of this technique to hVSMCs in culture. Of the two hVSMCs in this field, one is stained positively for bromodeoxyuridine incorporation (the nucleus is stained red) while the other cell shows staining only with the counterstain. Interestingly, autoradiographic detection of the labeled estradiol is noted only over the cell nucleus that is *negative* for BrdU incorporation.

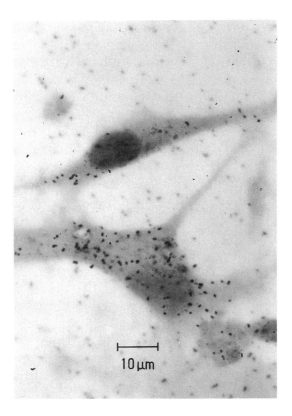

Figure 4 Double-labeling of cultured hVSMCs for bromodeoxyuridine incorporation and ER expression. Cell in upper left is stained positive for BrdU incorporation (red staining of nucleus) but shows little evidence of ^{3}H estradiol binding. Cell in lower right is negative for BrdU incorporation but does demonstrate significant autoradiographic evidence of ^{3}H estradiol binding, manifest as black grains surrounding nucleus, suggesting the presence of ER.

Thus, there is a dissociation of ER expression and evidence of proliferation. The hVSMC that is expressing ER shows no evidence of proliferative activity in this case. While these studies are ongoing in our laboratory, this is evidence of a possible relationship between ER expression and proliferative activity of hVSMCs in culture.

Five observations can be made from these data. First, serum containing high levels of estradiol induces significantly less proliferative activity of hVSMCs than does serum with low levels of estradiol. Second, the enhanced proliferation associated with low-E_2 serum is reduced by the addition of estradiol to this same serum. Third, there is a dose-response relationship between increasing concentrations of estradiol present in culture medium and decreasing proliferative activity of hVSMCs. Fourth, addition of specific ER antagonists to the culture medium before estradiol-containing serum blunts the antiproliferative effects of estradiol, suggesting that the antiproliferative effect of estradiol is a receptor-mediated phenomenon. Finally, in individual hVSMCs there is an apparent inverse relationship between ER expression and evidence of proliferative activity. These data support the notion that the effect of E_2 not only is mediated by the concentration of the ligand present, but may also be significantly affected by the level of expression of ER. Our preliminary data examining postmortem coronary arteries suggested, in fact, that diminished ER expression was associated with the development of coronary atherosclerosis in premenopausal women.

A principal finding of these studies is that of a clearly identified direct effect of estrogen on hVSMC behavior. By changing the concentration of estrogen in the cell-culture medium, thymidine incorporation was consistently and significantly altered. The absence of other cell types that could mediate the E_2 effect supports the notion that this effect is the result of direct interaction of estrogen with ER on the hVSMC. To ensure that the suppression of thymidine uptake by addition of E_2 to the culture medium was not a toxic effect, sample wells of all treated cells were subcultured after 72 hours and returned to a standard defined culture medium. Cell viability was shown to be equal in all treatment groups at this time point (data not shown). This indicates that E_2 is suppressive rather than toxic to hVSMCs.

With the above data as a background, demonstrating 1) evidence of ER expression in hVSMCs and 2) an antiproliferative effect of E_2 on ER-expressing populations of hVSMCs, our laboratory has now commenced examination of potential mechanisms by which E_2 could exert its antiproliferative effect.

I. Differential mRNA Expression by Genetically Identical hVSMCs in the Presence and Absence of Estrogen

The differential display of mRNA using the polymerase chain reaction is a recently described technique (79,80) used to identify and isolate genes that are differentially expressed in various cells under altered conditions. This technique uses a set of oligonucleotide primers, one of which is anchored to the polyadenylate tail of the mRNA while the other is short and arbitrary in sequence. The second primer is designed to anneal at different positions relative to the first primer. A reverse transcription reaction then results in the production of a subpopulation of complementary DNAs defined by these primers. The cDNAs are then amplified by polymerase chain reaction and resolved on a DNA-sequencing gel.

This technique is ideally suited to cell culture since the cells in culture, when they are derived from a single source, are genetically identical and differences in mRNA expression can therefore be ascribed to changing culture conditions. Our laboratory has begun using this technique to define the differences in gene expression that result when hVSMCs are exposed to estrogen in culture. There is a great degree of similarity in the amplified cDNA sequences defined on this gel. One particular band is present only in the lane corresponding to mRNA derived from hVSMCs exposed to female serum. This band is absent from lanes corresponding to cells exposed to male serum or female serum when these cells have been pretreated with an ER antagonist. The band is also absent from lanes corresponding to cells exposed to male or female serum that had been dextran charcoal-stripped. The differences in the cDNA defined on the sequencing gel correspond to differences in mRNA expression by hVSMCs when exposed to estrogen in female serum.

XI. SUMMARY

1.   Our laboratory has confirmed the expression of functional estrogen receptors in human vascular smooth muscle cells. Further evidence suggests a link between diminished ER expression and a propensity to coronary atherosclerosis.

2.   Evidence from our laboratory has also documented an antiproliferative effect of estrogen in the form of human female serum, as exogenous estrogen added to human male serum or added to charcoal-stripped fetal calf serum in defined culture media. The antiproliferative effect of estrogen appears to be unaltered by the presence of progesterone. Evidence for a receptor-mediated action of estrogen on hVSMCs is provided by the response of these cells to pretreatment with a pure ER antagonist (ICI 182780) before addition of estradiol (either endogenously contained in the serum of premenopausal women or exogenously added to male serum or charcoal-stripped fetal bovine serum). These findings suggest that both the estrogen content of the serum and the nature of the hVSMCs themselves are critical in the translation of E_2 effects on hVSMC biology.

3.   Evidence from our laboratory has also demonstrated a differential in mRNA expression in hVSMCs growing in the presence or absence of estrogen. Characterization of the changes in mRNA expression associated with E_2–ER binding and decreased proliferation will result in a clearer understanding of the mechanisms by which estrogen exerts a *direct* atheroprotective effect.

Coronary heart disease is the leading cause of death among postmenopausal women. This is in stark contrast to the relative freedom from coronary disease enjoyed by most premenopausal women. Elucidation of the effect of estrogen on vascular smooth muscle will provide important insights into the atherosclerotic disease process itself, as well as the opportunity to understand how best to extend the protection enjoyed by premenopausal women to women in older age groups, as well as to the male population.

REFERENCES

1. Bush TL, Miller VT. Effects of pharmacologic agents used during menopause: impact on lipids and lipoproteins. In: Mishell DR, ed. Menopause: Physiology and Pharmacology. Chicago: Year Book Medical Publishers, 1987:187–208.
2. Levy H, Boas EP. Coronary artery disease in women. JAMA 1936; 107:97.
3. Glendy RE, Levine SA, White PD. Coronary disease in youth: comparison of 100 patients under 40 with 300 persons past 80. JAMA 1937; 109:1775–1778.
4. Master AM, Dack S, Jaffe HL. Age, sex and hypertension in myocardial infarction due to coronary occlusion. Arch Intern Med 1939; 64:767.
5. Clawson BJ. The incidence of types of heart disease among 30,265 autopsies, with special reference to age and sex. Am Heart J 1941; 22:607.
6. Underdahl LO, Smith HL. Coronary artery disease in women under the age of 40. Proc Staff Meet Mayo Clin 1947; 22:479.
7. Rivan AU, Dimitroff SP. The incidence and severity of atherosclerosis in estrogen-treated males, and in females with a hypoestrogenic or a hyperestrogenic state. Circulation 1954; 9:533–539.
8. Oliver MF, Boyd GS. Effect of bilateral ovariectomy on coronary-artery disease and serum-lipid levels. Lancet 1959; ii:690–694.
9. Robinson RW, Higano N, Cohen WD. Increased incidence of coronary heart disease in women castrated prior to the menopause. Arch Intern Med 1959; 104:908–913.
10. Wuest JH, Dry TJ, Edwards JE. The degree of coronary atherosclerosis in bilaterally oophorectomized women. Circulation 1953; 7:801–808.
11. Ritterband AB, Jaffe IA, Densen PM, Magagna JF, Reed E. Gonadal function and the development of coronary heart disease. Circulation 1963; 27:237–251.

12. Novack ER, William TJ. Autopsy comparison of cardiovascular changes in castrated and normal women. Am J Obstet Gynecol 1966; 80:863–872.

13. Matthews KA, Meilahn E, Kuller LH, Kelsey SF, Caggiula AW, Wing RR. Menopause and risk factors for coronary heart disease. N Engl J Med 1989; 321:641–646.

14. Gurchow HW, Anderson AJ, Barboriak JJ, Sobocinski KA. Post-menopausal use of estrogen and occlusion of coronary arteries. Am Heart J 1988; 115:954–963.

15. Nabulsi AA, Folsom AR, White A, et al. Association of hormone-replacement therapy with various cardiovascular risk factors in postmenopausal women. N Engl J Med 1993; 328:1069–1075.

16. Knopp RH. Cardiovascular effects of endogenous and exogenous sex hormones over a woman's lifetime. Am J Obstet Gynecol 1988; 158:1630–1643.

17. Fischer GM, Swain ML. Effect of sex hormone on blood pressure and vascular connective tissue in castrated and noncastrated male rats. Am J Physiol 1977; 232:H617–H621.

18. Wolinsky H. Effects of estrogen and progestogen treatment on the response of the aorta of male rates to hypertension: Morphological and chemical studies. Circ Res 1972; 30:341–349.

19. Williams JK, Adams MR, Klopfenstein HS. Estrogen modulates responses of atherosclerotic coronary arteries. Circulation 1990; 81:1680–1687.

20. Kushwaha RS, Lewis DS, Carey KD, McGill HC Jr. Effects of estrogen and progesterone on plasma lipoproteins and experimental atherosclerosis in the baboon (Papio sp.). Arterioscler Thromb 1991; 11:23–31.

21. Tikkanen MJ, Nikkilä EA, Kuusi T, Sipinen S. High density lipoprotein$_2$ and hepatic lipase: reciprocal changes produced by estrogen and norgestrel. J Clin Endocrinol Metab 1982; 54:1113–1117.

22. Tikkanen MJ, Kuusi T, Nikkilä EA, Stenman U-H. Variation of postheparin plasma hepatic lipase by menstrual cycle. Metabolism 1986; 35:99–104.

23. Pick R, Stamler J, Rodbard S, Katz LN. The inhibition of coronary atherosclerosis by estrogen in cholesterol-fed chicks. Circulation 1952; 6:276–280.

24. Stamler J, Pick R, Katz LN. Prevention of coronary atherosclerosis by estrogen-androgen administration in the cholesterol-fed chick. Circ Res 1953; 1:94–98.

25. Adams MR, Kaplan JR, Koritnik DR, Clarkson TB. Pregnancy-associated inhibition of coronary artery atherosclerosis in monkeys: evidence of a relationship with endogenous estrogen. Arteriosclerosis 1987; 7:378–383.

26. Pick R, Stamler J, Rodbard S, Katz LN. Estrogen-induced regression of coronary atherosclerosis in cholesterol-fed chicks. Circulation 1952; 6:858–861.

27. Barrett-Connor E, Wingard DL, Criqui MH. Postmenopausal estrogen use and heart disease risk factors in the 1980s. JAMA 1989; 261:2095–2100.

28. Bush TL, Barrett-Connor E, Cowan LD. Cardiovascular mortality and non-contraceptive estrogen use in women: results from the Lipid Research Clinics' Program Follow-up Study. Circulation 1987; 75:1002–1009.

29. Reynolds SRM, Foster FI. Peripheral vascular action of estrogen, observed in the ear of the rabbit. J Pharmacol Exp Ther 1940; 68: 173–184.

30. Silva de Sá MF, Meirelles RS. Vasodilation effect of estrogen on the human umbilical artery. Gynecol Invest 1977; 8:307–313.

31. Williams JK, Adams MR, Herrington DM, Clarkson TB. Short-term administration of estrogen and vascular responses of atherosclerotic coronary arteries. JACC 1993; 20:452–457.

32. Maddox YT, Falcon JG, Ridinger M, Cunard CM, Ramwell PW. Endothelium-dependent gender differences in the response of the rat aorta. J Pharmacol Exp Ther 1987; 240:392–395.

33. Reis SE, Gloth ST, Blumenthal RS, et al. Ethinyl estradiol acutely attenuates abnormal coronary vasomotor responses to acetylcholine in postmenopausal women. Circulation 1994; 89:52–60.

34. Gilligan DM, Badar DM, Panza JA, Quyyumi AA, Cannon RO. Acute vascular effects of estrogen in postmenopausal women. Circulation 1994; 90:786–791.

35. Nichols NR, Olsson CA, Funder JW. Steroid effects on protein synthesis in cultured smooth muscle cells from rat aorta. Endocrinology 1983; 113:1096–1101.

36. Horwitz KB, Horwitz LD. Canine vascular tissues are targets for androgens, estrogens, progestins, and glucocorticoids. J Clin Invest 1982; 69:750–758.

37. Harder DR, Coulson PB. Estrogen receptors and effects of estrogen on membrane electrical properties of coronary vascular smooth muscle. J Cell Physiol 1979; 100:375–382.

38. Nakao J, Chang W-C, Murota S-I, Orimo H. Estradiol-binding sites in rat aortic smooth muscle cells in culture. Am Heart J 1981; 13767:12336–13364.

39. Colburn P, Buonassisi V. Estrogen-binding sites in endothelial cell cultures. Science 1978; 201:817–819.

40. Ricciardelli C, Horsfall DJ, Skinner JM, Henderson DW, Marshall VR, Tilley WD. Development and characterization of primary cultures of smooth muscle cells from the fibromuscular stroma of the guinea pig prostate. In Vitro Cell Dev Biol 1989; 25:1016–1024.

41. Elam MB, Lipscomb GE, Chesney CM, Terragno DA, Terragno NA. Effect of synthetic estrogen on platelet aggregation and vascular release of PGI_2-like material in the rabbit. Prostaglandins 1980; 20:1039–1051.

42. Kakar SS, Sellers JC, Devor DC, Musgrove LC, Neill JD. Angiotensin II type-1 receptor subtype cDNAs: differential tissue expression and hormonal regulation. Biochem Biophys Res Commun 1992; 183:1090–1096.

43. Green S. Promiscuous liaisons. Nature 1993; 361:590–591.

44. Green S, Chambon P. Nuclear receptors enhance our understanding of transcription regulation. Trends Genet 1988; 4:309–314.

45. Luisi BF, Xu WX, Otwinowski Z, Freedman LP, Yamamoto KR, Sigler PB. Crystallographic analysis of the interaction of the glucocorticoid receptor with DNA. Nature 1991; 352:497–505.

46. Carlberg C, Bendik I, Wyss A, et al. Two nuclear signalling pathways for vitamin D. Nature 1993; 361:657–660.

47. Jensen EV, Desombre ER. Mechanism of action of the female sex hormones. Annu Rev Biochem 1972; 41:203–230.

48. King WJ, Greene GL. Monoclonal antibodies localize estrogen receptor in the nuclei of target cells. Nature 1984; 307:745–747.

49. Welshons WV, Lieberman ME, Gorski J. Nuclear localization of unoccupied estrogen receptors. Nature 1984; 307:747–749.

50. Spelsburg TC, Webster RA, Pikler GM. Chromosomal proteins regulate steroid binding to chromatin. Nature 1976; 262:65–67.

51. Barrack ER, Coffey DS. The specific binding of estrogen and androgens to the nuclear matrix of sex hormone responsive tissues. J Biol Chem 1980; 255:7265–7275.

52. Pardoll DM, Vogelstein B, Coffey DS. A fixed site of DNA replication in eucaryotic cells. Cell 1980; 19:527–530.

53. Robinson SI, Nelkin BD, Vogelstein B. The ovalbumin gene is

associated with the nuclear matrix of chicken oviduct cells. Cell 1985; 28:99–106.

54. Walter P, Green S, Greene G, et al. Cloning of the human estrogen receptor cDNA. Proc Natl Acad Sci USA 1985; 82:7889–7893.

55. Aitken SC, Lippman ME. Hormonal regulation of *de novo* pyrimidine synthesis and utilization in human breast cancer cells in tissue culture. Cancer Res 1983; 43:4681–4690.

56. Aitken SC, Lippman ME. Effect of estrogens and antiestrogens on growth-regulatory enzymes in human breast cancer cells in tissue culture. Cancer Res 1985; 45:1611–1620.

57. Dickson RB, Lippman ME. Control of human breast cancer by estrogen, growth factors, and oncogenes. In: Lippmann ME, Dickson RB, eds. Breast Cancer: Cellular and Molecular Biology. Norwell, MA: Kluwer Academic Publishers, 1988:119–165.

58. Cowan K, Levine R, Aitken S, et al. Dihydrofolate reductase gene amplification and possible rearrangement in estrogen-responsive methotrexate resistant human breast cancer cells. J Biol Chem 1982; 257:15079–15086.

59. Kasid A, Davidson N, Gelmann E, Lippman ME. Transcriptional control of thymidine kinase gene expression by estrogens and antiestrogens in MCF-7 human breast cancer cells. J Biol Chem 1986; 261:5562–5567.

60. Stack G, Gorski J. Direct mitogenic effect of estrogen on the prepuberal rat uterus: studies on isolated nuclei. Endocrinology 1984; 115:1141–1150.

61. Sirbasku DA. Estrogen induction of growth factors specific for hormone-responsive mammary, pituitary, and kidney tumor cells. Proc Natl Acad Sci USA 1978; 75:3786–3790.

62. Sporn MB, Todaro GJ. Autocrine secretion and malignant transformation of cells. N Engl J Med 1980; 303:878–882.

63. Ma ZQ, Spreafico E, Pollio G, et al. Activated estrogen receptor mediates growth arrest and differentiation of a neuroblastoma cell line. Proc Natl Acad Sci USA 1993; 90:3740–3744.

64. Bradshaw MS, Tsai SY, Leng XH, et al. Studies on the mechanism of functional cooperativity between progesterone and estrogen receptors. J Biol Chem 1991; 266:16684–16690.

65. Jeng MH, Parker CJ, Jordan VC. Estrogenic potential of progestine in oral contraceptives to stimulate human breast cancer cell proliferation. Cancer Res 1992; 52:6539–6546.

66. Coibion M, Kiss R, Jossa V, et al. In vitro influence of estradiol or progesterone on the thymidine labeling indices of human benign breast tumors. Anticancer Res 1989; 9:475–482.
67. Scheven BA, Damen CA, Hamilton NJ, Verhaar HJ, Duursma SA. Stimulatory effects of estrogen and progesterone on proliferation and differentiation of normal human osteoblast-like cells in vitro. Biochem Biophys Res Commun 1992; 186:54–60.
68. Caronti B, Palladini G, Bevilacqua MG, et al. Effects of 17 beta-estradiol, progesterone and tamoxifen on in vitro proliferation of human pituitary adenomas: correlation with specific cellular receptors. Tumour Biol 1993; 14:59–68.
69. Michna H, Nishino Y, Neef G, McGuire WL, Schneider MR. Progesterone antagonists: tumor-inhibiting potential and mechanism of action. J Steroid Biochem Mol Biol 1992; 41:339–348.
70. Okulicz WC, Balsamo M, Tast J. Progesterone regulation of endometrial estrogen receptor and cell proliferation during the late proliferative and secretory phase in artificial menstrual cycles in the rhesus monkey. Biol Reprod 1993; 49:24–32.
71. Losordo DW, Kearney M, Kim EA, Jekanowski J, Isner JM. Variable expression of the estrogen receptor in normal and atherosclerotic coronary arteries of premenopausal women. Circulation 1994; 89:1501–1510.
72. Pickering JG, Weir L, Rosenfield K, Stetz J, Jekanowski J, Isner JM. Smooth muscle cell outgrowth from human atherosclerotic plaque: implications for the assessment of lesion biology. J Am Coll Cardiol 1992; 20:1430–1439.
73. Horwitz KB, Costlow ME, McGuire WL. MCF-7: a human breast cancer cell line with estrogen, androgen, progesterone, and glucocorticoid receptors. Steroids 1975; 26:785–795.
74. Karas RH, Patterson BL, Mendelsohn ME. Human vascular smooth muscle cells contain functional estrogen receptor. Circulation 1994; 89:1943–1950.
75. Klein-Hitpass L, Kaling M, Ryffel GU. Synergism of closely adjacent estrogen-responsive elements increases their regulatory potential. J Mol Biol 1988; 201:537–544.
76. Klein-Hitpass L, Ryffel GU, Heitlinger E, Cato AC. A 13 bp palindrome is a functional estrogen responsive element and interacts specifically with estrogen receptor. Nucleic Acids Res 1988; 16: 647–663.
77. Hiort O, Kwan PWL, DeLellis RA. Immunohistochemistry of es-

trogen receptor protein in paraffin sections: effects of enzymatic pretreatment and cobalt chloride intensification. Am J Clin Pathol 1988; 90:559–563.

78. Rutqvist LE, Mattsson A. Cardiac and thromboembolic morbidity among postmenopausal women with early-stage breast cancer in a randomized trial of adjuvant tamoxifen. J Natl Cancer Inst 1993; 85:1398–1406.

79. Liang P, Pardee AB. Differential display of eukaryotic messenger RNA by means of the polymerase chain reaction. Science 1992; 257:967–971.

80. Liang P, Averboukh L, Pardee AB. Distribution and cloning of eukaryotic mRNA's by means of differential display: refinements and optimization. Nucleic Acids Res 1993; 21:3269–3275.

3

The Epidemiology of Menopause and Its Association with Cardiovascular Disease

Jan A. Staessen, Leszek Bieniaszewski, Ivo Brosens, and Robert Fagard

University of Leuven
Leuven, Belgium

I. INTRODUCTION

The climacteric, a normal aging phenomenon in women, is the gradual transition from the reproductive to the nonreproductive phase of life (1). The menopause is usually defined as the cessation of menstruation (2) or the last menstrual period (1) and marks the end of ovulation. The onset of relative infertility antedates menopause by a variable period of 5 to 10 years (1).

Ovarian failure following the menopause is characterized by estrogen deficiency. Estrogens may exert a powerful protective effect on the cardiovascular system, for instance, by increasing the ratio of high-density to low-density lipoproteins in plasma (3) or by inhibiting arterial vasomotion (4,5) and thrombosis (6). From a hemodynamic point of view, premenopausal women have a higher resting heart rate, cardiac index, and pulse pressure, but a lower total peripheral resistance than men with a similar mean arterial pressure (7). Other studies have shown that at submaximal exercise, women achieve the same oxygen uptake as men despite a lower stroke volume as a result of a more pronounced increase in heart rate and oxygen extraction (8). These gender differences disappear after menopause (7).

From an epidemiological point of view, most (1,9–24), although not all (25–34), reports have demonstrated an increased incidence of cardiovascular diseases after menopause. Despite the vast literature already available, the influence of menopause on the cardiovascular system—in particular, on the pathogenesis of hypertension—remains debated. The main reason for this is the difficulty of separating the effects of menopause per se from those of aging and other factors related to the aging process. This chapter reviews the epidemiology of menopause and its relationship with cardiovascular disease, in particular, hypertension and coronary heart disease. The intervention studies, in which estrogens were administered to postmenopausal subjects, are discussed in Chapter 10, and are therefore summarized here only to the extent that they are helpful in understanding the observational epidemiological reports.

II. MENOPAUSE

A. Mechanism

The mechanism underlying menopause is the disappearance of the ovarian follicles (35). This process starts before birth, continues through the reproductive phase of life, and terminates during the climacterium and the perimenopausal period (36). With advancing age, the remaining ovarian follicles become less sensitive to gonadotropins and secrete less estrogen. As a consequence, the serum concentration of follicle-stimulating hormone rises, the normal peak of luteinizing hormone in the blood disappears (37), and the menstrual cycle becomes anovulatoric. After menopause, progesterone is only produced by the adrenals in a nonpulsating pattern, and the dominant estrogen is not estradiol. Instead, estrone is produced by the peripheral conversion in adipose tissue of androstenedione, secreted by the adrenals (38,39). However, after menopause, the adrenal production of androstenedione falls and the circulating androstenedione is roughly only half that secreted before menopause (40). Thus, after menopause, estrogen deficiency prevails.

B. Age at Menopause

The distribution of menopausal age is negatively skewed (1). Under these circumstances, the use of mean age at menopause gives excessive weight to the wide scatter of precocious menopausal age, thereby underestimating the true average age at menopause. Median age should therefore be used to describe the central tendency of the distribution of menopausal age (1).

Retrospective interviews tend to underestimate the age at menopause because, due to digit preference, women tend to round up the recollected age of menopause to 40, 45, or 50 years (35). Even in prospective studies menopause is variously defined as beginning with the last episode of bleeding, or after amenorrhea has been present for 9 months or longer. Nevertheless, there is striking concordance among most studies (1,41–49) that in Western industrialized societies the median age at the menopause is currently around 50 years (Table 1). In non-Caucasian women, however, the menopause seems to occur earlier. American (48) and South African (50) black women have an earlier menopause than their white counterparts. Moreover, malnutrition and low body weight are associated with a precocious menopause (35).

The most important factor determining a woman's age at the menopause is the number of ovarian follicles (35). Human primordial germ cells separate from the somatic cells at an early stage of embryogenesis. Some 1000 to 2000 migrate to the gonadal

Table 1 Age at Menopause Reported by Several Investigators

Study	Country	Median age[a]	Mean age[b]
Benjamin, 1960 (41)	South Africa (whites)	50.0	48.7
von Hauser and Wenner, 1961 (46)	Israel	—	49.5
Frommer, 1964 (43)	United Kingdom	50.1	50.8
MacMahon and Worcester, 1966 (48)	United States	49.8	47.3
Burch and Gunz, 1967 (42)	New Zealand	50.7	—
Jaszmann et al., 1969 (44)	The Netherlands	—	51.4
McKinlay et al., 1972 (45)	United Kingdom	50.8	47.5
Treloar, 1974 (47)	United States	49.8	—
Lindquist, 1982 (1)	Sweden	50.4	49.1
Staessen et al., 1989 (83)	Belgium	—	53.0

[a]Age at which half the women had reached menopause.
[b]Arithmetic mean, which may underestimate the central tendency of the distribution of age at menopause (see text for further explanation).

ridge, where they rapidly multiply to up to 5 to 7 million follicles around the fifth month of intrauterine life. Thereafter, multiplication ceases and the primordial follicles commence to dissolve, so that at birth both fetal ovaries combined contain no more than about 2 million follicles (51,52). This number continues to fall after birth. Fewer than 0.02% of the follicles present at birth are ovulated during the reproductive phase of life; the remainder degenerate. In the immediate premenopausal period, the rate of loss of primordial follicles accelerates, and menopause intervenes when the number of follicles has fallen below a critical number (53,54).

Nulliparous women tend to have an earlier menopause (41,55), while increased parity, particularly in higher social classes, is associated with a later menopause (45,56). Mothers of twins enter the menopause about 1 year earlier than women who have only had singleton infants (56). Women whose last pregnancy occurred before the age of 28 probably have an earlier menopause than those with the last pregnancy at a later age (57). Blindness may also lead to a later menopause, which suggests that the pineal gland may play a role in maintaining the menstrual cycle (58). With the exception of mumps oophoritis, pelvic or systemic infections rarely cause ovarian failure (35).

Women who smoke enter the menopause up to 2 years earlier than those who do not (59–61). The effects of smoking on the age at menopause seem to be dose-related and may be mediated partly through a lowered estrogen production (62–65). Moreover, tobacco smoke contains toxic and carcinogenic substances, which may potentially contribute to the premature aging and destruction of primordial oocytes in the ovaria (66).

C. The Social Impact of Menopause

By the year 2025, 23% of the population will be aged 60 or over. As a result of the increasing life expectancy in the First and Second Worlds, many women will be postmenopausal for over one-third of their lives (67). Already, approximately 95% of all women living in industrialized countries experience menopause during their lifetime (68). These numbers help to explain why over the past decades menopause has grown from a subject peripheral to medical interest into one that takes a central place in clinical practice and about which there is a lively debate both in medical journals and in the lay press (2).

III. HYPERTENSION

Systolic pressure increases with age at least until the eighth decade of life (69–71), whereas diastolic pressure rises only until 50 years of age (Figure 1). Following middle age, both systolic and diastolic blood pressure become higher in women than in men, whereas the reverse is true in the first half of life. This observation suggests that ovarian failure and the ensuing estrogen deficiency may influence the age-related increase in blood pressure in women. However, the blood-pressure changes associated with menopause are difficult to evaluate, because menopause coincides with aging, and because both menopause and blood pressure are influenced by such factors as body mass index (1,72), socioeconomic class (73,74), and smoking (59–61,75,76).

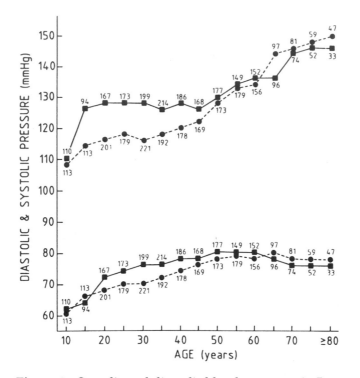

Figure 1 Systolic and diastolic blood pressures in 5-year age classes in a representative sample (n = 4202) of the population of five Belgian districts. In each subject, five blood-pressure readings were obtained at each of two home visits. The five blood-pressure readings from the second home visit were averaged for this presentation. For each sex (■ men, n = 2044; ● women, n = 2158) and age group, the number of subjects contributing to the mean is given (From Ref. 71.)

Taylor et al. (77) were among the first to contrast the prevalence of hypertension in menopausal women and office workers. They found that hypertension was no more common in a group of 179 castrated women and 21 women with natural menopause than in the control subjects and that "vasomotor instability," as exhibited by hot flashes, perspiration, and tachycardia, was not necessarily associated with hypertension (77). The obvious conclusion from this pioneering study (77) was that the relationship between hypertension and menopause was incidental and that the loss of ovarian secretion was neither a primary nor a contributory cause of arterial hypertension.

Since these early observations (77), several longitudinal (78–82) and cross-sectional (11,72,73,83,84) studies have addressed the alleged association between hypertension and menopause. However, their conclusions remain contradictory (Table 2).

A. Longitudinal Studies

In Framingham, Hjortland et al. (78) followed for nine biannual examinations a cohort of 1686 middle-aged women, who were premenopausal at the initial examination. Of these, 480 became menopausal, 77 underwent hysterectomy without oophorectomy or with just unilateral oophorectomy, and 137 were subjected to bilateral oophorectomy. The blood-pressure changes in these women were compared with those observed in 3117 controls. The Framingham team found that menopause was not accompanied by significant changes in blood pressure (Table 2), body weight, and blood glucose, whereas hemoglobin rose in the postmenopausal women (78,85). However, women undergoing spontaneous menopause were significantly leaner than their controls. Thus, the menopausal subjects in the Framingham cohort (78) differed from their premenopausal counterparts in more aspects than just menstrual status.

Lindquist et al. (1,10,72,79) published several reports on the influence of menopause on cardiovascular risk profile. In a cohort study, 1263 women from 38 to 54 years old at the initial examination were followed for 6 years. Women whose amenorrhea at the follow-up examination had lasted less than 6 months, women taking estrogens, and women in whom the menopause had been surgically or radiologically induced were excluded from the analysis. Of the remaining 973 women, 326 stayed premenopausal through the 6 years of follow-up, 343 passed through menopause with amenorrhea persisting for at least 6 months, and 304 were postmenopausal both at the start and at the end of follow-up.

Table 2 Association Between Menopause and Blood Pressure in Various Studies

Study	Type of menopause[a]	Adjustments[b]	ΔSBP	ΔDBP	HT[c]
Longitudinal					
Hjortland et al., 1976 (78)	N (480) vs. P (3117)	MT, A	−0.8c	−0.2c	
	H (77) vs. P (3117)	MT, A	−0.3c	+1.4c	
	C (137) vs. P (3117)	MT, A	−0.1c	−0.6c	
Linquist, 1982 (79)	N (343) vs. P (324)	A	−1.1c	−1.0c	
	N (343) vs. P (304)	A	+0.1c	+0.9c	
van Berensteyn et al., 1989 (81)	N (168)	BMI, IA, IBP, IBMI	−1.3d	−0.6d	
van Berensteyn et al., 1992 (82)	N (37)	BMI, IA, IBP, IBMI	−0.7d	−0.1d	
	N (139)	BMI, IA, IBP, IBMI	−0.7d	−0.2d	
	N (63)	BMI, IA, IBP, IBMI	+1.1d	−0.3d	
Cross-sectional					
Weiss, 1972 (11)	N (297), S (172), P (428)	A	+4.7c	+2.7c	
Lindquist and Bengtsson, 1980 (72)	N (162) vs. P (164), 50 years old	A	−5.0c	0c	
Eferakeya and Imasuen, 1986 (73)	N (681) vs. P (728), other ages	A	−5.4c	−1.1c	
	N (287) vs. P (252)	A, SEC	+16.1c	+15.7c	
Staessen et al., 1989 (83)	N and S (120 and 64) vs. P (278)	A, AHT, BMI, EP, PR	+0.5e	+2.5c	+30 (>140/>90)
Wu et al., 1990 (84)	N (176) vs. P (422)	A	+2.9c	−0.1c	+8 (>140/>90)
Other designs					
Taylor et al., 1947 (77)	N and C (21 and 179) vs. OW (2860)				−1 (>149/>94)

[a]C = castrated women (bilateral oophorectomy); H = women who underwent hysterectomy not combined with bilateral oophorectomy; N = women with natural menopause; OW = office workers; P = premenopausal (control) subjects; S = women who underwent surgical menopause.

[b]A = age; AHT = antihypertensive treatment; BMI = body mass index; EP = intake of estrogens and/or progestogens; IA = initial age; IBP = initial blood pressure; IBMI = initial body mass index; MT = measurement technique; PR = pulse rate; SEC = socioeconomic class.

[c]ΔSBP, ΔDBP = change in systolic, diastolic pressure (mm Hg) associated with menopause, taken directly from the publications or calculated according to the published results with weighting by number, if the published articles included more than 1 group; HT = difference in the prevalence of hypertension (percent) as defined by the systolic/diastolic blood pressure criteria (mm Hg) given in parentheses.

[d]Age-related changes (mm Hg/yr) in various groups of menopausal women.

[e]Difference in slope of systolic pressure on age associated with menopause (mm Hg/yr).

Weight gain was observed in the women who remained premenopausal throughout follow-up (+2.2 kg) and in those who stopped menstruating (+1.5 kg), but not in subjects who were already postmenopausal at entry into the study (+0.4 kg). Systolic and diastolic pressure rose with age, but the age-related blood-pressure increases were similar in the three groups of women (Table 2) (79). There was also no increased need for antihypertensive treatment in women who had experienced a change in their menstrual status during follow-up.

In a population-based study in Ede, in The Netherlands, the blood pressure of healthy perimenopausal women, who were 49–56 years old at the initial examination, was followed annually for 10 years (81,82,86,87). A major limitation of this survey was the important selection at recruitment, which renders generalizations difficult. All women (n = 4,018) born between 1922 and 1931 were asked to participate, but only 402 (10%) responded. Moreover, participation in this survey was limited by the investigators to those women who were not on medication known to influence blood pressure, calcium metabolism, or the time of onset of menopause (e.g., steroids, antihypertensive agents, or insulin), and to those who did not have a history of hypertension, major gynecological surgery, or serious diseases of the kidney or bone tissue. On the basis of these eligibility criteria, 209 of the 402 respondents were immediately excluded.

A first report covered 7 years of follow-up in the Ede survey (81) and included 168 of the 193 selected respondents, i.e., 4% of all subjects invited. A total of 19 participants had dropped out and six were excluded from the analysis, because the onset of menopause could not be determined as a result of estrogen substitution. The analysis was carried out following a complex mixed-longitudinal approach (86,87), which, according to the authors, made it possible to separate how aging and menopause per se had affected blood pressure. In the 168 women, body weight rose by only 0.15 kg per year and blood pressure did not increase. In multivariate analyses, systolic as well as diastolic pressure showed a significant negative relationship (slope, −1.34 and −0.63 mm Hg per year, respectively) with the years since menopause. On the other hand, the observed positive relationship (slope, 0.81 mm Hg per year) of systolic pressure with chronological aging was not significant, nor was a consistent association found between diastolic pressure and chronological aging. The latter observations, which are at variance with the usual epidemiological experience in Western communities, are probably reflective of the high degree of selection involved in recruiting the participants into the Ede survey. Nevertheless, from this first report, van Beresteyn et al. (81) concluded that menopause should not be regarded as a possible cause of hypertension.

The full 10-year follow-up experience in the Ede survey was published later in a second report (82), which now included 167 women. For the statistical analysis, this time the total person-time experience was subdivided into three menopausal periods. Based on years relative to menopause, three menopausal cohorts were created starting 2 years before ($n = 37$), 2 years after ($n = 139$), and 6 years after menopause ($n = 63$). Each group had been followed for 4 years. The longitudinal design of the survey provided an opportunity to study not only the "natural history" of blood pressure, but also the effects of dietary calcium during and after the period of ovarian failure. The habitual calcium intake, estimated by dietary history, averaged 1110 mg per day, varying from 560 to 2580 mg per day. Changes in systolic and diastolic blood pressure during the menopausal periods were adjusted for the concurrent alterations in body mass index and other relevant variables. An average decline in systolic pressure by 6 mm Hg was observed from 2 years before to 6 years after menopause, and an increase of almost 5 mm Hg from 6 to 10 years after menopause. A significant change in diastolic pressure was not observed (Table 2). Neither changes in, nor the absolute level of, calcium intake showed any relevant association with blood-pressure change. The conclusions drawn after 10 years of follow-up of the selective Ede cohort were therefore that 1) ovarian failure seemed to temporarily reverse the increase in blood pressure due to aging and 2) a habitual calcium intake exceeding 800 to 1000 mg per day was not effective in preventing hypertension in the postmenopausal period (82).

In a prospective study of 468 middle-aged normotensive women (systolic/diastolic pressure <140/90 mm Hg) (80), the behavioral and biological predictors of a blood-pressure increase from baseline to the follow-up examination 3 years later were evaluated. The participation rate in this study was 60% (541 of 901 invited women), and 73 subjects were excluded from the analysis. The factors, which were significantly and independently associated with a rise in systolic pressure, included increased anger and anxiety scores on standardized psychological tests, a higher fasting insulin at baseline, a parental history of hypertension, and increases in body mass index and alcohol intake over the 3 years of follow-up. A rise in diastolic pressure was related to being black, and to increases in body mass index, hematocrit, and anger scores and decreases in the dietary intake of potassium. Menopausal status and hormone-replacement therapy were unrelated to the changes in blood pressure in this report (80), but the exact quantitative influence of menopausal status on blood pressure, adjusted for confounders, was not presented.

B. Cross-Sectional Studies

Weiss (11) examined in a cross-sectional study 897 women who were selected from the United States Health Examination Survey (1960–1962). Women whose menstrual periods had stopped had higher levels of serum cholesterol and diastolic blood pressure (Table 2) than premenopausal women. For systolic pressure a similar tendency was present in three of four age classes. In the postmenopausal women, serum cholesterol and blood-pressure levels were not related to the type of menopause (spontaneous vs. operative) or to the time interval since menopause. Weiss concluded from his observations that menopause probably preceded the rises in serum cholesterol and diastolic blood pressure. More recently, the results from the second National Health and Nutrition Examination Survey (1976–1980) (88) showed that, after adjusting for age, body size, smoking, oral contraceptive use, education, poverty status, and alcohol consumption, systolic pressure was inversely associated with gravidity in both premenopausal and postmenopausal subjects. The partial regression coefficients (± standard error) were compatible with a decrease in systolic pressure, averaging 0.47 ± 0.21 mm Hg per pregnancy before menopause and 0.39 ± 0.17 mm Hg per pregnancy after menopause.

In 50-year-old women studied cross-sectionally in 1968 and 1969, Lindquist and Bengtsson (72) found that systolic pressure was on average 5 mm Hg (p <0.05) higher in 164 premenopausal women than in 162 postmenopausal subjects, whereas their diastolic pressure was the same (Table 2). The premenopausal women were also 3.7 kg (p <0.001) heavier than their postmenopausal counterparts, which could explain the higher systolic pressure in the former. In the women of the other age strata (44 to 56 years), there were no systematic blood-pressure differences according to menstrual status, but the number of pre- and postmenopausal women within each of these strata was largely dissimilar, which made the comparisons less reliable than in the 50-year-old group.

Eferakeya and Imasuen (73) examined in a cross-sectional study 539 Nigerian women, from 35 to 54 years old, of whom 252 were premenopausal, 152 had not menstruated for 6 to 11 months (menopausal subjects), and 135 had ceased to menstruate for 12 months at least (postmenopausal subjects). The menopausal and postmenopausal women had higher systolic and diastolic pressures than their age-matched premenopausal controls, irrespective of socioeconomic class (Table 2). In this cross-sectional survey in Benin (Africa) (73), all blood-pressure readings were taken by the same observer, but this researcher was probably not blinded with respect to the menstrual status of the participants.

In Belgium, the association between menopause and systolic and diastolic blood pressure was explored in a random sample of 278 pre- and 184 postmenopausal women, who were from 35 to 59 years old (83). In 64 of the postmenopausal subjects, menopause had been surgically induced. All women were participants in a Belgian cross-sectional population survey with a sample size of 3950 eligible persons, of whom 67% took part. All subjects in the survey were characterized by the average of 10 blood-pressure readings, i.e., five consecutive readings in the sitting position obtained at each of two home visits. In the Belgian study, a self-administered questionnaire was used to evaluate menstrual status, lifestyle (74), and the intake of medications. Natural menopause was defined as the reported cessation of periods and surgical menopause as the disappearance of menstruation following a gynecological operation.

In the Belgian survey (83), the postmenopausal women had higher systolic (132 vs. 121 mm Hg), diastolic (81 vs. 75 mm Hg), and pulse (51 vs. 46 mm Hg) pressures than the premenopausal subjects (Figure 2). Hypertension, defined as being on antihypertensive medication—regardless of the blood-pressure level—or as having a blood pressure exceeding 140 mm Hg systolic or 90 mm Hg diastolic, was more frequently observed following menopause (40 vs. 10%; p <0.001). After stratification by age and body mass index, the odds of having hypertension in premenopausal as compared with postmenopausal women were 2.2 (95% confidence interval from 1.1 to 4.4; p = 0.03). After adjustment of blood pressure for significant covariates, such as body mass index, pulse rate, and the intake of estrogens and/or progestogens, the slope of systolic pressure on age was 0.5 mm Hg per year steeper in all women with natural and surgical menopause than in the premenopausal subjects (Figure 3). The relationship of diastolic pressure to age had the same slope in pre- and postmenopausal subjects, but in women with natural and surgical menopause, taken together, the regression line was shifted upward by an average of 2.3 mm Hg (p = <0.03). The relationship of diastolic pressure to body mass index and to the urinary sodium:potassium ratio were also 2.0 mm Hg per kg/m^2 and 0.8 mm Hg per unit steeper (p = <0.05) in postmenopausal than in premenopausal subjects.

In a recent Asian study, the blood pressure was measured in 598 Chinese women from 40 to 54 years old (84). The women were categorized into three groups: 1) premenopausal women (n = 176), 2) menopausal women, who had menstruated irregularly for at least 6 months or who had not menstruated for 11 months (n = 193), and 3) postmenopausal women, who had ceased to menstruate for at least 12 months and who had not had hysterectomy (n = 229). The blood pressure of each subject was measured twice by two physicians simultaneously. The average

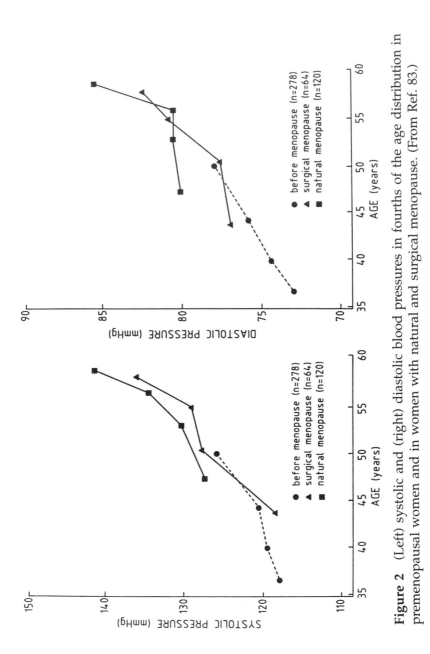

Figure 2 (Left) systolic and (right) diastolic blood pressures in fourths of the age distribution in premenopausal women and in women with natural and surgical menopause. (From Ref. 83.)

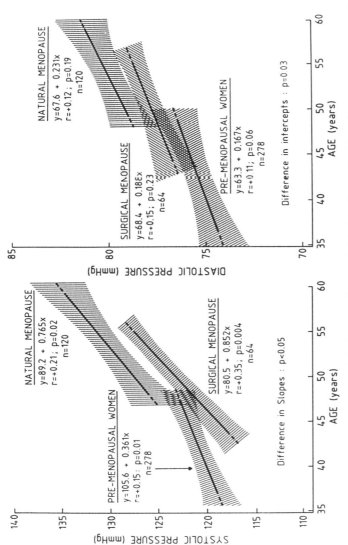

Figure 3 Regression lines of (left) systolic and (right) diastolic blood pressure on age in premenopausal women ($n = 278$) and in subjects with natural ($n = 120$) or surgical ($n = 64$) menopause. The regression lines were standardized for body mass index (26.6 kg/m²), pulse rate (74 beats per minute), the urinary sodium:potassium ratio (2.4), intake of estroprogestogens (none), and antihypertensive treatment (none). (From Ref. 83.)

of all these blood-pressure readings was used for analyzing and estimating the prevalence of hypertension and hypotension. Hypertension was defined according to the usual World Health Organisation criteria (89). Hypotension was a systolic pressure less than 90 mm Hg or a diastolic pressure less than 60 mm Hg or both. Women who had been diagnosed as hypertensive and who were taking antihypertensive drugs during the period of examination were always classified as hypertensive, regardless of their blood pressure. In this Chinese study (84), systolic and diastolic blood pressure were on average the same in the three groups differentiated according to menstrual status (Table 2). However, after stratification for age, menopausal and postmenopausal women, compared with premenopausal subjects, showed higher prevalences of definite hypertension (18 and 21%, respectively, vs. 12%), borderline and definite hypertension combined (24 and 23% vs. 19%) and hypotension (15 and 4% vs. 1%) (84).

C.   Hypertension Related to Menopause: A Plausible Working Hypothesis?

On balance, the longitudinal surveys (78,79,81,82) suggest that menopause per se is not associated with an increase in blood pressure and a greater incidence of hypertension. The results from the cross-sectional studies are more equivocal (Table 2), as some surveys (11,73,83) have found a positive association and other studies no relationship (72,84). Although longitudinal studies are often considered to be superior to cross-sectional surveys, both are open to confounding. Cross-sectional designs may preclude the accurate assessment of changes over time, due to differences in growth or development across generations (cohort differences). Longitudinal surveys, on the other hand, are easily confounded by effects related to the time of measurement. Changes in the environmental conditions inevitably occur over a given period of follow-up, and may lead to an over-or underestimation of the true intraindividual changes and relationships over time (86). In particular, clinical, biochemical, and technical measurements may be unduly influenced by the unavoidable renewal of chemicals, standards, and instrumentation, or by changes in the team of observers.

Both cross-sectional (11,72,73,83,84) and longitudinal (78, 79,81,82) observational studies have their limitations. Moreover, reports on estrogen-substitution therapy after menopause (see below) have convincingly demonstrated that correction of the postmenopausal estrogen deficiency is accompanied by a decrease in the incidence of cardiovascular complications. One is therefore left with the possibility that the rise in systolic pressure following menopause may be due at least in part to menopause per se. Measurement of blood pressure by new methods, which are less subject to observer bias (90,91), may help to clarify this situation in the near future.

Several possible mechanisms come to mind to explain the alleged increase in blood pressure following menopause. Menopause is accompanied by weight gain (79,83,92) and a rise in the circulating insulin levels (80). The postmenopausal estrogen deficiency may affect the balance between various vasoactive hormones (93,94) and the proliferation (95) and function (4,5) of vascular smooth-muscle cells, possibly by altering the electrolyte composition of the intra-cellular (93) or extracellular (96,97) milieu. Menopause, through a redistribution of body sodium and the cessation of periods, is followed by a rise in hemoglobin and in the erythrocyte count (78), thereby increasing blood viscosity, and in turn possibly blood pressure as well (76,98). In a Dutch study (12), menopause has also been found to be associated with calcification of the abdominal aorta. After adjustment for age and other cardiovascular risk indicators, women with natural menopause had a 3.4 times greater risk of having atherosclerosis of the abdominal aorta than premenopausal subjects (95% confidence interval: 1.2 to 9.7; $p < 0.05$), and women with surgical menopause a 5.5 greater risk (1.9 to 15.8; $p < 0.005$). Stiffening of the large arteries after menopause may explain why, as observed in the Belgian survey (83), the slope of systolic pressure on age steepened and the pulse pressure widened in the postmenopausal subjects.

IV.   OTHER CARDIOVASCULAR DISEASES

In premenopausal women, the prevalence and incidence of cardiovascular diseases are lower than in middle-aged men. The
cardiovascular risk of women rises after the age of 50, although
even in postmenopausal women the incidence of fatal and nonfatal cardiovascular complications combined still remains nearly
45% lower than in age-matched male subjects (99). Nevertheless,
in absolute numbers, more women then men die from cardiovascular illnesses at an older age, because the aged female population at risk is substantially larger than the male.

A.   The Association Between Menopause and Cardiovascular Disease

The relationship between menopause and cardiovascular disease—in particular, ischemic heart disease—has been examined
in several studies, of which most (1,10,14–24), but not all (26–34),
found that the age-adjusted rates rose after menopause.

   In Göteborg, Sweden, for people 45 to 54 years of age, the
incidence of myocardial infarction was six times higher in men
than in women (1,100). However, the prevalence of angina pectoris, as determined from a questionnaire, was similar in both
sexes (1). The higher case-fatality rate of myocardial infarction in
the Swedish men probably explained to some extent the lack of a
sex difference in the occurrence of angina pectoris (1).

   According to an early report on the Framingham Study
(101), among the subjects younger than 60 years of age with
primary uncomplicated angina pectoris, 35% of the men, but only
15% of the women, died within 8 years. Thus, being female
seemed to confer a protective effect against ischemic heart disease (101). In more recent reports on the Framingham Study
(17,25), the relationship between menopause and the incidence of
cardiovascular disease was further explored in women who were
less than 55 years old and who had been drawn from the initial
2873 female participants enrolled int he Framingham cohort (25).
The number of person-years during the 20 years of follow-up

was nearly the same among the pre- and postmenopausal subjects. Nevertheless, there were only 20 cardiovascular events in the former, whereas 70 events occurred in the postmenopausal subjects (25). In each age group studied, the incidence of cardiovascular events was lower in premenopausal than in postmenopausal women. This was also true for coronary heart disease. The contrast according to menstrual status for "hard" diagnoses of cardiovascular disease—thus excluding diagnoses of angina pectoris and intermittent claudication—was in the same direction. Although cholesterol and hemoglobin did slightly rise in women undergoing menopause, the greater incidence of cardiovascular disease in the postmenopausal Framingham women could not be explained by the influence of menopause on the usual cardiovascular risk factors (25).

The Nurses' Health Study (9) included 121,700 American women from 30 to 55 years old, who were followed from 1976 to 1982. In this prospective cohort study (9), the relationship between menopause and the risk of coronary heart disease was studied. Information on menopausal status, the type of menopause, and other risk factors was first collected in 1976 and updated every 2 years by mailing questionnaires. Through 1982, the follow-up rate was 98% for mortality and 95% for nonfatal events. After adjustment for age and cigarette smoking, women who had undergone a natural menopause and who had never taken estrogen-replacement therapy, had no appreciable increase in the risk of coronary heart disease, as compared with premenopausal women (adjusted rate ratio; 1.2; 95% confidence limits: 0.8 and 1.8). Again compared with premenopausal women, the occurrence of a natural menopause together with the use of estrogens did not affect the coronary risk (rate ratio: 0.8; 95% confidence limits: 0.4 and 1.3). By contrast, women who had undergone bilateral oophorectomy and who had never taken estrogens after menopause had an increased risk (rate ratio: 2 2; 95% confidence limits: 1.2 and 4.2). However, the use of estrogens in the postmenopausal period appeared to eliminate this augmented risk as compared with the premenopausal subjects (rate ratio: 0.9; 95% confidence limits: 0.6 and 1.6). This large cohort study (9) therefore suggested that, unlike natural menopause, bilateral oophorectomy raised the risk of coronary heart disease, but that this increased risk could be reversed by estrogen-replacement therapy. On the other hand, the findings of the Nurses' Health Study were gathered in a highly educated and health-conscious professional group and are therefore not necessarily applicable to the population at large.

B. Is the Association Between Menopause and Cardiovascular Disease Causal?

The issue of whether ovarian failure is to blame for the loss of female protection from cardiovascular disease after the menopause is difficult to answer. The incidence of cardiovascular disease rises with age without abrupt increase after menopause, so, exactly as for hypertension, the effects of menopause per se and aging are extremely difficult to separate. However, several lines of evidence suggest that menopause on its own may be involved in explaining the higher cardiovascular morbidity and mortality in postmenopausal compared with premenopausal subjects.

If estrogens protect the cardiovascular system from complications, an acute alteration in the risk following the menopause should not be expected, because the circulating estrogen levels decline slowly in the perimenopausal phase of follicular senescence. In a cohort study spanning a follow-up of 2 years (102), serum low-density lipoprotein cholesterol and total cholesterol rose significantly and high-density lipoprotein cholesterol declined in women who became menopausal, compared with the cohort members who aged similarly but still menstruated. The lipid values at baseline were already less favorable in the subjects who subsequently became menopausal. The latter observations (102) and other studies (1,10,11,72,73,78,79,84,85,103,104) suggest that the cardiovascular risk profile—in particular, the serum lipid levels (Figure 4)—deteriorate gradually during the perimenopausal years.

In women who underwent bilateral oophorectomy at an early age and in whom ovarian failure is abruptly induced, the

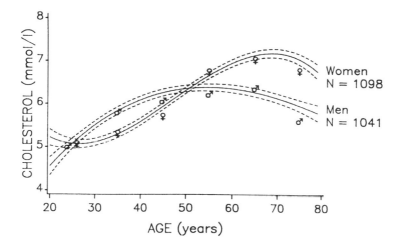

Figure 4 Total serum cholesterol in a representative sample ($n = 2139$) of the population of two Belgian districts. For each sex, symbols represent the average cholesterol values in 10-year age classes. The regression lines with 95% confidence intervals were calculated from data in individual subjects.

incidence of cardiovascular disease is substantially higher than in menstruating women of similar age (9,13,14,16,18,20,24,25,105, 106). A plausible explanation for these observations is that the changes in the circulating estrogen levels in castrated women are acute and therefore more readily visible in terms of cardiovascular complications.

Estrogens directly influence several cardiovascular risk factors, whereby the greatest weight is usually given to the changes in the serum lipid and lipoprotein concentrations (107–111). In general, estrogens raise the serum level of high-density lipoprotein cholesterol, especially the HDL_2 subfraction, and lower the serum concentration of low-density lipoprotein cholesterol (107–112). Usually, estrogens also produce a slight decrease in serum total cholesterol. These are the theoretically desirable changes cited most frequently to support the epidemiological findings pertaining to estrogen deficiency and cardiovascular disease

(107–112). Oral estrogens also elevate serum triglyceride concentrations, but this is not considered an important adverse effect (110). On the other hand, the lipid changes associated with menopause may not necessarily be applicable to all races, because in a case-control study in American Pima Indians including 148 premenopausal and 75 age-matched postmenopausal women, menopause was not associated with an increase in the serum concentration of total cholesterol (113). However, in both Pima men and women, total serum cholesterol was 20 to 30% lower than in white subjects and also did not increase with advancing age (113).

Retrospective evidence from case-control (114–123) and other (124) studies of postmenopausal women treated with estrogens, mostly unopposed conjugated equine estrogens, in general support or at least do not contradict the concept of a cardioprotective effect of estrogen (Table 3). In many of the case-control studies (114,117,123), relatively few women treated with estrogens were included (16% on average) and the duration of treatment was short (15 months). These factors probably explain why the benefit of estrogen-replacement therapy was significant in only one of the case-control studies (118). Another single study (116), which had recruited many young smoking women, seemed to negate the protective effect of exogenous estrogen-replacement therapy. In contrast, most of the prospective but nonrandomized cohort studies of estrogen therapy in postmenopausal women (125–135) indicate a clear benefit in terms of coronary artery disease and show a lower mortality from coronary and cardiovascular complications (Table 3).

V. GENERAL CONCLUSIONS

Menopause, i.e., the end of menstruation, constitutes an important physiological and psychological change in a women's life time and usually takes place at around 50 years of age (Table 1). Systematic interest in the menopause by physicians arose in the middle of the last century, at a time when the interest in the care

Table 3 Association Between Hormone-Replacement Therapy and Ischemic Heart Disease

Study	No. of cases[a]	Relative risk[b]
Case-control		
Adam et al., 1981 (120)	76 (151)	E: 0.7
Bain et al., 1981 (199)	123 (2460)	C: 0.7, E: 0.9
Jick et al., 1978 (116)	17 (34)	C: 7.5
Pfeffer et al., 1978 (115)	196 (520)	C: 0.8, E: 0.9
Szklo et al., 1984 (121)	39 (45)	E: 0.6
Rosenberg et al., 1976 (114)	366 (6830)	C: 1.0
Rosenberg et al., 1980 (117)	447 (1832)	C: 1.3, F: 1.2
Ross et al., 1981 (118)	133 (266)	Vs. living controls—E: 0.4; vs. dead controls—E: 0.6
Thompson et al., 1989 (123)	603 (1206)	E: 1.4[c]
Cohort		
Bush et al, 1987 (132)	50 (2270)	Fatal CHD—C: 0.4
Burch et al., 1974 (125)	9 (737)	Fatal CHD—C: 0.4
Criqui et al., 1988 (134)	87 (1868)	Fatal CHD—0.8
Hammond et al., 1979 (128)	58 (610)	CHD—C: 0.3
Henderson et al., 1991 (133)	149 (8841)	Fatal MI—C: 0.6 <> fatal CHD—C: 0.8
Hunt et al., 1987 (131)	20 (4544)	Fatal CHD—C: 0.5
Petitti et al., 1979 (126)	26 (16,759)	MI—C: 1.2
Petitti et al., 1986 (127)	37 (16,638)	Fatal CVD—E: 0.5
Stampfer et al., 1985 (130)	90 (32,317)	Fatal and nonfatal CHD—C: 0.3, E: 0.5
Stampfer et al., 1991 (135)	205 (48,470)	CHD—C: 0.6, F: 0.8; fatal CVD—C: 0.6, F: 0.8
Wilson et al., 1985 (129)	48 (1234)	CHD—C: 1.9; fatal CVD—C: 1.9

[a]Number of controls or total number of subjects enrolled in the cohort studies is in parentheses.
[b]Risk of ischemic heart disease in women who received estrogen-replacement therapy vs. women who did not. C = risk ratio for users vs. nonusers or never-users; E = risk ratio for ever-users vs. never-users; F = risk ratio for former users vs. never-users. CHD = coronary heart disease; CVD = cardiovascular disease; MI = myocardial infarction.
[c]Strokes ($n = 244$) and myocardial infarctions ($n = 359$) were combined.

of the "diseases of women" grew exponentially (2). However, it is only in the last decades of the 20th century that the postmenopausal years have become generally recognized as a phase of the female life cycle that in some of its aspects may benefit from medical intervention (2).

Despite these new insights, it remains extremely difficult to disentangle the effects of aging and menopause per se on the cardiovascular system, on the recognized cardiovascular risk indicators, and on the prevalence and incidence of cardiovascular illnesses, such as hypertension and coronary heart disease. For instance, epidemiological observations on their own could not establish with certainty that menopause is independently associated with a raised cardiovascular risk. This became unambiguously clear only after the cohort studies (Table 3) had overwhelmingly demonstrated that estrogen-replacement therapy is accompanied by a decrease in overall mortality, which is mediated principally through a beneficial effect on the incidence and fatality rate of coronary heart disease (125–135).

The protective effect of exogenous estrogens in postmenopausal women (3,6,67,107,111,112,136) strongly suggests that ovarian failure, in its own right, must constitute a cardiovascular risk factor. Estrogen deficiency may principally, albeit not exclusively, operate through its influence on the lipid metabolism. Also, other cardiovascular risk factors, such as obesity (1,72) and blood viscosity (76,98), are altered in an unfavorable way following menopause.

The influence of menopause per se on blood pressure, a major cardiovascular risk factor in older persons (137), remains uncertain. The cohort studies (78,79,81,82) do not support a direct influence of menopause on the incidence of hypertension, and the evidence from the cross-sectional studies (11,72,73,83,84) is equivocal. Nevertheless, there is some suggestion that estrogen-replacement treatment may reduce the incidence of stroke (128). One may therefore envisage the possibility that observational studies with more bias-free methods to measure the blood pressure than conventional sphygmomanometry, such as ambulatory monitoring (138–141), as well as further studies with estrogen-replacement therapy will tilt the alleged positive association between menopause and blood-pressure elevation above the horizon of epidemiological visibility.

ACKNOWLEDGMENTS

Epidemiological research relevant to this chapter has been supported by the International Lead Zinc Research Organization (Research Triangle Park, North Carolina), the Province of Limburg (Hasselt, Belgium), the municipalities Hechtel-Eksel and Lommel (Belgium), the National Fund for Medical Research, the Incentive Program *Health Hazards* (Science Policy Office, Prime Minister's Services), the Ministry of the Flemish Community (Department of Labor and Social Affairs), Astra Pharmaceuticals Inc., Bristol-Meyers Squibb Inc. (all in Brussels, Belgium), and Schwarz Pharma AG (Mannheim, Germany). The secretarial assistance of Mrs. I. Tassens is gratefully acknowledged.

REFERENCES

1. Lindquist O. Influence of the menopause on ischaemic heart disease and its risk factors and on bone mineral content. Acta Obstet Gynecol Scand 1982; 110(suppl):7–32.
2. Lock M. Contested meanings of the menopause. Lancet 1991; 337:1270–1272.
3. Ayalon D, Pines A. Cardiovascular disease and hormone replacement therapy: a review. Isr J Med Sci 1993; 29:660–663.
4. Sarrel PM. Ovarian hormones and the circulation. Maturitas 1990; 12:287–298.
5. Gangar KF, Vyas S, Whitehead M, Crook D, Meire H, Campbell S. Pulsatility index in internal carotid artery in relation to transdermal oestradiol and time since menopause. Lancet 1991; 338: 839–842.
6. Ettinger B. Hormone replacement therapy and coronary heart disease. Obstet Gynecol Clin North Am 1990; 17:741–757.

7. Messerli FH, Garavaglia GE, Schmieder RE, Sundgaard-Riise K, Nunez BD, Amodeo C. Disparate cardiovascular findings in men and women with essential hypertension. Ann Intern Med 1987; 107:158–161.

8. Fagard RH, Thijs LB, Amery AK. The effect of gender on aerobic power and exercise hemodynamics in hypertensive adults. Med Sci Sports Exercise 1994; 27:29–34.

9. Colditz GA, Willett WC, Stampfer MJ, Rosner B, Speizer FE, Hennekens CH. Menopause and the risk of coronary heart disease in women. N Engl J Med 1987; 316:1105–1110.

10. Lindquist O, Bengtsson C, Lapidus L. Relationships between the menopause and risk factors for ischaemic heart disease. Acta Obstet Gynecol Scand 1985; 130:43–47.

11. Weiss NS. Relationship of menopause to serum cholesterol and arterial blood pressure: the United States Health Examination Survey of Adults. Am J Epidemiol 1972; 96:237–241.

12. Witteman JCM, Grobbee DE, Kok FJ, Hofman A, Valkenburg HA. Increased risk of atherosclerosis in women after the menopause. Br Med J 1989; 298:642–644.

13. Higano N, Robinson RW, Cohen WD. Increased incidence of cardiovascular disease in castrated women: Two-year follow-up studies. Med Intelligence 1995; 268:1123–1125.

14. Wuest JH Jr, Dry TJ, Edwards JE. The degree of coronary atherosclerosis in bilaterally oophorectomized women. Circulation 1953; 7:801–808.

15. Johansson S, Vedin A, Wilhelmsson C. Myocardial infarction in women. Epidemiol Rev 1983; 5:67–95.

16. Oliver MF, Boyd GS. Effect of bilateral ovariectomy on coronary-artery disease and serum-lipid levels. Lancet 1959; ii:690–694.

17. Gordon T, Kannel WB, Hjortland MC, McNamara PM. Menopause and coronary heart disease: the Framingham Study. Ann Intern Med 1978; 89:157–161.

18. Brinkley D, Haybittle JL. The late effects of artificial menopause by X-radiation. Br J Radiol 1969; 42:519–521.

19. Rosenberg L, Hennekens CH, Rosner B, Belanger C, Rothman KJ, Speizer FE. Early menopause and the risk of myocardial infarction. Am J Obstet Gynecol 1981; 139:47–51.

20. Novac ER, Williams TJ. Autopsy comparison of cardiovascular changes in castrated and normal women. Am J Obstet Gynecol 1960; 80:863–872.

21. Bengtsson C. Ischaemic heart disease in women: a study based on a randomized population sample of women and women with myocardial infarction in Göteborg, Sweden. Acta Med Scand 1973; 549(suppl):1–128.

22. Winkelstein W, Jr., Stenchever MA, Lilienfeld AM. Occurrence of pregnancy, abortion, and artificial menopause among women with coronary heart disease: a preliminary study. J Chronic Dis 1958; 7:273–286.

23. Spitzer RS, Lee KT, Thomas WA. Early age of menopause in young women with fatal acute myocardial infarction. Am Heart J 1957; 53:805–808.

24. Parrish HM, Carr CA, Hall DG, King TM. Time interval from castration in premenopausal women to development of excessive coronary atherosclerosis. Am J Obstet Gynecol 1967; 99: 155–162.

25. Kannel WB, Hjortland MC, McNamara PM, Gordon T. Menopause and risk of cardiovascular disease: The Framingham Study. Ann Intern Med 1976; 85:447–452.

26. Heller RF, Jacobs HS. Coronary heart disease in relation to age, sex, and the menopause. Br Med J 1978; 1:472–474.

27. Ritterband AB, Jaffe IA, Densen PM, Magagna JF, Reed E. Gonadal function and the development of coronary heart disease. Circulation 1963; 27:237–251.

28. Alderson MR, Jackson SM. Long term follow-up of patients with menorrhagia treated by irradiation. Br J Radiol 1971; 44:295–298.

29. Randall CL, Paloucek FP, Graham JB, Graham S. Causes of death in cases of preclimacteric menorrhagia. Am J Obstet Gynecol 1964; 88:880–897.

30. Wilhelmsen L, Bengtsson C, Elmfeldt D, et al. Multiple risk prediction of myocardial infarction in women as compared with men. Br Heart J 1977; 39:1179–1185.

31. Mulcahy R, Hickey N, Maurer B. Coronary heart disease in women: study of risk factors in 100 patients less than 60 years of age. Circulation 1967; 36:577–586.

32. Mann JI, Doll R, Thorogood M, Vessey MP, Waters WE. Risk factors for myocardial infarction in young women. Br J Prev Soc Med 1976; 30:94–100.

33. Manchester JH, Herman MV, Gorlin R. Premenopausal castration and documented coronary atherosclerosis. Am J Cardiol 1971; 28:33–37.

34. Blanc JJ, Boschat J, Morin JF, Clavier J, Penther P. Menopause and myocardial infarction. Am J Obstet Gynecol 1977; 127:353–355.
35. Ginsburg J. What determines the age at the menopause? The number of ovarian follicles seems the most important factor. Br Med J 1991; 302:1288–1289.
36. Sherman BM, West JH, Korenman SG. The menopausal transition: analysis of LH, FSH, estradiol, and progesterone concentrations during menstrual cycles of older women. J Clin Endocrinol Metab 1976; 629–636.
37. Judd HL, Shamonki IM, Frumar AM, Lagasse LD. Origin of serum estradiol in postmenopausal women. Obstet Gynecol 1982; 59:680–686.
38. Grodin JM, Siiteri PK, MacDonald PC. Source of estrogen production in postmenopausal women. J Clin Endocrinol Metab 1973; 36:207–214.
39. Horton R, Tait JF. Androstenedione production and interconversion rates measured in peripheral blood and studies on the possible site of its conversion to testosterone. J Clin Invest 1966; 45:301–313.
40. Meldrum DR, Davidson BJ, Tataryn IV, Judd HL. Changes in circulating steroids with aging in postmenopausal women. Obstet Gynecol 1981; 57:624–628.
41. Benjamin F. The age of the menarche and of the menopause in white South African women and certain factors influencing these times. S Afr Med J 1960; 34:316–320.
42. Burch PRJ, Gunz FW. The distribution of the menopausal age in New Zealand: An exploratory study. NZ Med J 1967; 6:6–10.
43. Frommer DJ. Changing age of the menopause. Br Med J 1964; 2:349–351.
44. Jaszmann L, van Lith ND, Zaat JCA. The age at menopause in The Netherlands: The statistical analysis of a survey. Int J Fertil 1969; 14:106.
45. McKinlay S, Jefferys M, Thompson B. An investigation of the age at menopause. J Biosoc Sci 1972; 4:161–173.
46. von Hauser GA, Wenner R. Das Klimakterium der Frau. Ergeb Inn Med Kinderheilkd 1961; 125–168.
47. Treloar AE. Menarche, menopause and intervening fecundability. Hum Biol 1974; 89–107.
48. MacMahon B, Worcester J. Age at menopause: United States. Government Printing Office, Washington, DC: U.S. Department

of Health, Education and Welfare, Public Health Service, National Center for Health Statistics, 1966.

49. Treloar AE. Menstrual cyclicity and the pre-menopause. Maturitas 1981; 3:249–264.
50. Frere G. Mean age at menopause and menarche in South Africa. S Afr Med J 1971; 36:21–24.
51. Block E. Quantitative morphological investigations of the follicular system in women. Acta Anat (Basel) 1952; 14:108–123.
52. Baker TG. A quantitative and cytological study of germ cells in human ovaries. Proc R Soc Lond (Biol) 1963; 158:417–433.
53. Richardson SJ, Senikas V, Nelson JF. Follicular depletion during the menopausal transition: evidence for accelerated loss and ultimate exhaustion. J Clin Endocrinol Metab 1987; 65:1231–1237.
54. Richardson SJ, Nelson JF. Follicular depletion during the menopausal transition. Ann NY Acad Sci 1990; 592:13–20.
55. von Hauser GA, Remen U, Valaer M, Erb H, Müller T, Orbiri J. Menarche and menopause in Israel. Gynaecologia (Basel) 1963; 155:39–47.
56. Soberon J, Calderon JJ, Goldzieher JW. Relation of parity to age at menopause. Am J Obstet Gynecol 1966; 96–100.
57. Brand PG, Lehert PH. A new way of looking at environmental variables that may affect the age at menopause. Maturitas 1978; 1:121–132.
58. Lehrer S. Fertility and menopause in blind women. Fertil Steril 1981; 36:396–398.
59. Jick H, Porter J, Morrison AS. Relation between smoking and age of natural menopause: Report from the Boston Collaborative Drug Surveillance Program, Boston University Medical Center. Lancet 1977; i:1354–1355.
60. Andersen FS, Transböl I, Christiansen C. Is cigarette smoking a promotor of the menopause? Acta Med Scand 1982; 212:137–139.
61. Adena MA, Gallagher HG. Cigarette smoking and the age at menopause. Ann Hum Biol 1982; 9:121–130.
62. Khaw KT, Tazuke S, Barrett-Conner E. Cigarette smoking and levels of adrenal androgens in postmenopausal women. N Engl J Med 1988; 318:1705–1709.
63. Baron JA, Adams P, Ward M. Cigarette smoking and other correlates of cytologic estrogen effect in postmenopausal women. Fertil Steril 1988; 766–771.
64. Longcope C, Johnston CC Jr. Androgen and estrogen dynamics

in pre- and post-menopausal women: a comparison between smokers and non-smokers. J Clin Endocrinol Metab 1988; 67: 379–383.

65. Kaufman DW, Slone D, Rosenberg L, Miettinen OS, Shapiro S. Cigarette smoking and age at natural menopause. Am J Public Health 1980; 70:420–422.

66. Matisson DR, Thorgeirsson SS. Smoking and industrial pollution and their effects on menopause and ovarian cancer. Lancet 1978; i:187–188.

67. Sitruk-Ware R, Ibarra de Palacios P. Estrogen replacement therapy and cardiovascular disease in post-menopausal women: A review. Maturitas 1989; 11:259–274.

68. Zachariasen RD. Oral manifestations of menopause. Compend Contin Educ Dent 1995; 12:1584–1591.

69. Kannel WB, Gordon T. Evaluation of cardiovascular risk in the elderly: the Framingham Study. Bull NY Acad Med 1978; 54: 573–591.

70. Staessen J, Bulpitt C, Fagard R, Joossens JV, Lijnen P, Amery A. Four urinary cations and blood pressure: a population study in two Belgian towns. Am J Epidemiol 1983; 117:676–687.

71. Staessen J, Amery A, Fagard R. Editorial review: Isolated systolic hypertension in the elderly. J Hypertens 1990; 8:393–405.

72. Lindquist O, Bengtsson C. Serum lipids, arterial blood pressure and body weight in relation to the menopause: results from a population study of women in Göteborg, Sweden. Scand J Clin Lab Invest 1980; 40:629–636.

73. Eferakeya AE, Imasuen JE. Relationship of menopause to serum cholesterol and arterial blood pressure in some Nigerian women. Public Health 1986; 100:28–32.

74. Staessen JA, Fagard R, Amery A. Life style as a determinant of blood pressure in the general population. Am J Hypertens 1994; 7:685–694.

75. Staessen JA, Atkins N, Fagard R, O'Brien ET, Thijs L, Amery A. Correlates of the diurnal blood pressure profile in a population study. High Blood Press 1993; 2:271–282.

76. Chabanel A, Chien S. Blood viscosity as a factor in human hypertension. In: Laragh JH, Brenner BM, eds. Hypertension: Pathophysiology, Diagnosis, and Management. Vol 1. New York, Raven Press, 1990:329–337.

77. Taylor RD, Corcoron AC, Page IH. Menopausal hypertension: a critical study. Am J Med Sci 1947; 213:475–476.
78. Hjortland MC, McNamara PM, Kannel WB. Some atherogenic concomitants of menopause: the Framingham study. Am J Epidemiol 1976; 103:304–311.
79. Lindquist O. Intraindividual changes of blood pressure, serum lipids, and body weight in relation to menstrual status: results from a prospective population study of women in Göteborg, Sweden. Prev Med 1982; 11:162–172.
80. Markovitz JH, Matthews KA, Wing RR, Kuller LH, Meilahn EN. Psychological, biological and health behavior predictors of blood pressure changes in middle-aged women. J Hypertens 1991; 9:399–406.
81. van Beresteyn ECH, Van 't Hof MA, De Waard H. Contributions of ovarian failure and aging to blood pressure in normotensive perimenopausal women: a mixed longitudinal study. Am J Epidemiol 1989; 129:947–955.
82. van Beresteijn ECH, Riedstra M, Van der Wel A, Schouten EG, Burema J, Kok FJ. Habitual dietary calcium intake and blood pressure change around the menopause: a longitudinal study. Int J Epidemiol 1992; 21:683–689.
83. Staessen J, Bulpitt CJ, Fagard R, Lijnen P, Amery A. The influence of menopause on blood pressure. J Hum Hypertens 1989; 3: 427–433.
84. Wu Z, Wu X, Zhang Y. Relationship of menopausal status and sex hormones to serum lipids and blood pressure. Int J Epidemiol 1990; 19:297–302.
85. Thorell B, Svärdsudd K. Myocardial infarction risk factors and well-being among 50-year-old women before and after the menopause. Scand J Prim Health Care 1993; 11:141–146.
86. Van 't Hof MA, Roede MJ, Kowalski CJ. A mixed longitudinal data analysis model. Hum Biol 1977; 49:165–179.
87. van Beresteyn ECH, Van 't Hof MA, De Waard H, et al. Design and data quality of a mixed longitudinal study to elucidate the role of dietary calcium and phosphorus on bone mineralization in pre-, peri-, and postmenopausal women. Am J Clin Nutr 1986; 43:538–548.
88. Ness RB, Kramer RA, Flegal KM. Gravidity, blood pressure, and hypertension among white women in the Second National Health

and Nutrition Examination Survey. Epidemiology 1993; 4:303–309.

89. The Guidelines Subcommittee of the WHO/ISH Mild Hypertension Liaison Committee. 1993 guidelines for the management of mild hypertension. Memorandum from a World Health Organization/International Society of Hypertension Meeting. Hypertension 1993; 22:392–403.

90. Staessen J, O'Brien E, Atkins N, et al. The increase in blood pressure with age and body mass index is overestimated by conventional sphygmomanometry. Am J Epidemiol 1992; 136: 450–459.

91. Staessen JA, Fagard R, Lijnen P, et al. Ambulatory blood pressure and blood pressure measured at home: progress report on a population study. J Cardiovasc Pharmacol 1994; 23(suppl 5): S5–S11.

92. Wing RR, Matthews KA, Kuller LH, Meilahn EN, Plantinga PL. Weight gain at the time of menopause. Arch Intern Med 1991; 151:97–102.

93. M'Buyamba-Kabangu JR, Lijnen P, Fagard R, et al. Erythrocyte concentrations and transmembrane fluxes of sodium and potassium and biochemical measurements during the menstrual cycle in normal women. Am J Obstet Gynecol 1985; 151:687–693.

94. Sundsfjord JA, Aakvaag A. Plasma renin activity, plasma renin substrate and urinary aldosterone excretion in the menstrual cycle in relation to the concentration of progesterone and oestrogens in the plasma. Acta Endocrinol 1972; 71:519–525.

95. Fischer-Dzoga K, Wissler RW, Vesselinovitch D. The effects of oestradiol on the proliferation of rabbit aortic tissue culture cells induced by hyperlipemic serum. Exp Mol Pathol 1983; 39: 355–363.

96. Aitken JM, Lindsay R, Hart DM. The redistribution of body sodium in women on long-term oestrogen therapy. Clin Sci Mol Med 1974; 47:179–187.

97. Hodgkinson A. Plasma electrolyte concentrations in women and the effects of oestrogen administration. Maturitas 1982; 4:247–256.

98. Yarnell JWG, Baker IA, Sweetnam PM, et al. Fibrinogen, viscosity, and white blood cell count are major risk factors for ischemic heart disease. The Caerphilly and Speedwell Collaborative Heart Disease Studies. Circulation 1991; 83:836–844.

99. Bush TL. The epidemiology of cardiovascular disease in post-menopausal women. Ann NY Acad Sci 1990; 59:263–271.

100. Elmfeldt D, Wilhelmsen L, Tibblin G, Vedin JA, Wilhelmsson CE, Bengtsson C. Registration of myocardial infarction in the city of Göteborg, Sweden: A community study. J Chronic Dis 1975; 28:173–178.

101. Kannel WB, Feinleib M. Natural history of angina pectoris in the Framingham study: Prognosis and survival. Am J Cardiol 1972; 29:154–163.

102. Matthews KA, Meilahn E, Kuller LH, Kelsey SF, Caggiula AW, Wing RR. Menopause and risk factors for coronary heart disease. N Engl J Med 1989; 321:641–646.

103. Tominaga T, Suzuki H, Ogata Y, Matsukawa S, Saruta T. The role of sex hormones and sodium intake in postmenopausal hypertenson. J Hum Hypertens 1991; 5:495–500.

104. Shibata H, Matsuzaki T, Hatano S. Relationship of relevant factors of atherosclerosis to menopause in Japanese women. Am J Epidemiol 1979; 109:420–424.

105. Weiss NS. Premature menopause and aortoiliac occlusive disease. J Chronic Dis 1972; 25:133–138.

106. Ask-Upmark E. Life and death without ovaries. Acta Med Scand 1962; 172:129–135.

107. Belchetz PE. Hormonal treatment of postmenopausal women. N Engl J Med 1994; 330:1062–1071.

108. Rijpkema AHM, van der Sanden AA, Ruijs AHC. Effects of postmenopausal oestrogen-progestogen replacement therapy on serum lipids and lipoproteins: a review. Maturitas 1990; 12:259–285.

109. Lobo RA. Clinical review 27: effects of hormonal replacement on lipids and lipoproteins in postmenopausal women. J Clin Endocrinol Metab 1991; 73:925–930.

110. Walsh BW, Schiff I, Rosner B, Greenberg L, Ravnikar V, Sacks FM. Effects of postmenopausal estrogen replacement on the concentrations and metabolism of plasma lipoproteins. N Engl J Med 1991; 325:1196–1204.

111. Ravn SH, Rosenberg J, Bostofte E. Postmenopausal hormone replacement therapy—clinical implications. Eur J Obstet Gynecol Reprod Biol 1994; 53:81–93.

112. Knopp RH. Cardiovascular effects of endogenous and exogenous sex hormones over a women's lifetime. Am J Obstet Gynecol 1988; 158:1630–1643.

113. Hamman RF, Bennett PH, Miller M. The effect of menopause on serum cholesterol in American (Pima) Indian women. Am J Epidemiol 1975; 102:164–169.

114. Rosenberg L, Armstrong B, Jick H. Myocardial infarction and estrogen therapy in post-menopausal women. N Engl J Med 1976; 294:1256–1259.

115. Pfeffer RI, Whipple GH, Kurosaki TT, Chapman JM. Coronary risk and estrogen use in postmenopausal women. Am J Epidemiol 1978; 107:479–497.

116. Jick H, Dinan B, Rothman KJ. Noncontraceptive estrogens and nonfatal myocardial infarction. JAMA 1978; 239:1407–1408.

117. Rosenberg L, Slone D, Shapiro S, Kaufman D, Stolley PD, Miettinen OS. Noncontraceptive estrogens and myocardial infarction in young women. JAMA 1980; 244:339–342.

118. Ross RK, Paganini-Hill A, Mack TM, Arthur M, Henderson BE. Menopausal oestrogen therapy and protection from death from ischaemic heart disease. Lancet 1981; i:858–860.

119. Bain C, Willett W, Hennekens CH, Rosner B, Belanger C, Speizer FE. Use of postmenopausal hormones and risk of myocardial infarction. Circulation 1981; 64:42–46.

120. Adam S, Williams V, Vessey MP. Cardiovascular disease and hormone replacement treatment: a pilot case-control study. Br Med J 1981; 282:1277–1278.

121. Szklo M, Tonascia J, Gordis L, Bloom I. Estrogen use and myocardial infarction risk: a case-control study. Prev Med 1984; 13: 510–516.

122. Croft P, Hannaford PC. Risk factors for acute myocardial infarction in women: evidence from the Royal College of General Practitioners' oral contraceptive study. Br Med J 1989; 298:165–168.

123. Thompson SG, Meade TW, Greenberg G. The use of hormonal replacement and the risk of stroke and myocardial infarction in women. J Epidemiol Community Health 1989; 43:173–178.

124. Sullivan JM, Vander Zwaag R, Lemp GF, et al. Postmenopausal estrogen use and coronary atherosclerosis. Ann Intern Med 1988; 108:358–363.

125. Burch JC, Byrd BF Jr, Vaughn WK. The effects of long-term estrogen in hysterectomized women. Am J Obstet Gynecol 1974; 118:778–782.

126. Petitti DB, Wingerd J, Pellegrin F, Ramcharan S. Risk of vascular

disease in women: Smoking, oral contraceptives, noncontraceptive estrogens, and other factors. JAMA 1979; 242:1150–1154.

127. Petitti DB, Perlman JA, Sidney S. Postmenopausal estrogen use and heart disease. N Engl J Med 1986; 315:131–132.

128. Hammond CB, Jelovsek FR, Lee KL, Creasman WT, Parker RT. Effects of long-term estrogen replacement therapy. I. Metabolic effects. Am J Obstet Gynecol 1979; 133:525–536.

129. Wilson PWF, Garrison RJ, Castelli WP. Postmenopausal estrogen use, cigarette smoking, and cardiovascular morbidity in women over 50: The Framingham Study. N Engl J Med 1985; 313:1038–1043.

130. Stampfer MJ, Willett WC, Colditz GA, Rosner B, Speizer FE, Hennekens CH. A prospective study of postmenopausal estrogen therapy and coronary heart disease. N Engl J Med 1985; 313: 1044–1049.

131. Hunt K, Vessey M, McPherson K, Coleman M. Long-term surveillance of mortality and cancer incidence in women receiving hormone replacement therapy. Br J Obstet Gynaecol 1987; 94: 620–635.

132. Bush TL, Barrett-Connor E, Cowan LD, et al. Cardiovascular mortality and noncontraceptive use of estrogen in women: results from the Lipid Research Clinics' Program Follow-up Study. Circulation 1987; 75:1102–1109.

133. Henderson BE, Paganini-Hill A, Ross RK. Decreased mortality in users of estrogen replacement therapy. Arch Intern Med 1991; 151:75–78.

134. Criqui MH, Suarez L, Barrett-Connor E, McPhillips J, Wingard DL, Garland C. Postmenopausal estrogen use and mortality: results from a prospective study in a defined, homogeneous community. Am J Epidemiol 1988; 128:606–614.

135. Stampfer MJ, Colditz GA, Willett WC, et al. Postmenopausal estrogen therapy and cardiovascular disease: ten-year follow-up from the Nurses' Health Study. N Engl J Med 1991; 325:756–762.

136. Radwanska E. The role of reproductive hormones in vascular disease and hypertension. Steroids 1993; 58:605–610.

137. Staessen J, Amery A, Birkenhäger W, et al. Is a high serum cholesterol associated with longer survival in elderly hypertensives? J Hypertens 1990; 8:755–761.

138. The Scientific Committee. Consensus document on non-invasive

ambulatory blood pressure monitoring. J Hypertens 1990; 8(suppl 6):S135–S140.

139. Pickering TG, O'Brien ET. Second international consensus meeting on twenty-four-hour blood pressure measurement: consensus and conclusions. J Hypertens 1991; 9(suppl 8):S2–S6.

140. Pickering TG. The ninth Sir George Pickering memorial lecture ambulatory monitoring and the definition of hypertension. J Hypertens 1992; 10:401–409.

141. Mancia G, Bertinieri G, Grassi G, et al. Effects of blood pressure measurement by the doctor on patient's blood pressure and heart rate. Lancet 1983; ii:695–698.

4

Hemodynamics and Pathogenesis

Franz C. Aepfelbacher and Franz H. Messerli
Ochsner Clinic
New Orleans, Louisiana

I. INTRODUCTION

As many as 50% of all women in the Westernized world will develop high blood pressure during their lifetime. In the vast majority of cases, we are not able to determine a specific cause for this disorder and therefore classify these cases as "essential" or "primary." Sir George Pickering, after carefully reviewing the relationship between gender and prognosis for essential hypertension, concluded 40 years ago that "for any given high blood pressure at any age, women seem to fare better than men" (1). Data from the Framingham Heart Study clearly supported this hypothesis by showing that women have a markedly lower risk of cardiovascular disease as compared to men with the same level of arterial pressure (2–4). However, it is a well-known fact that women lose their resistance to cardiovascular disease with advancing age. A recent study from the Framingham cohort demonstrated the importance of menopausal status in the annual incidence of coronary heart disease (Figure 1) (5): Documented onset of menopause quadrupled the risk for a coronary event compared with women the same age who remained premenopausal.

In this chapter, we review the hemodynamic findings in essential hypertension, with special emphasis on gender differences and menopausal status of women, and give an overview of current pathogenetic concepts in this disorder.

II. HEMODYNAMIC PATTERNS OF HYPERTENSION

The two hemodynamic determinants of blood pressure are cardiac output and the peripheral resistance of the arteries, total

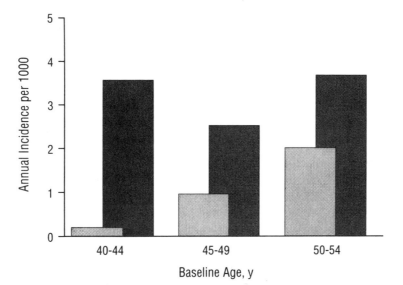

Figure 1   The annual incidence of coronary heart disease according to menopausal status at the biennial examination in women aged 40 to 54 years at study entry. Data are from the 18-year follow-up of the Framingham Study. Gray bars indicate premenopausal women; black bars, postmenopausal women. The overall risk is 4.17; p <0.001. (From Ref. 5.)

peripheral resistance (TPR). A dysproportional elevation of either of these factors will lead to hypertension; however, the hemodynamic alterations responsible for increased blood pressure vary, and depend on age, body weight, and stage of the hypertensive disease.

The characteristic hemodynamic disturbance in the younger patient with borderline or stage I hypertension is a high cardiac output and a numerically normal calculated TPR (6–8). In the presence of obesity, cardiac output is elevated even further and intravascular volume is expanded, which can actually lead to "low" calculated TPR (9). This stage of early hypertension is sometimes called the hyperkinetic phase, and there has been much debate about whether an increase in cardiac output might be responsible for a sustained increase in blood pressure in essential hypertension. However, hemodynamic studies during exercise in the early stage of hypertension revealed that TPR does not fall to the same extent as in normotensives, indicating that resistance vessels are affected even early in the course of hypertension (10).

As hypertension becomes more established, the dominating hemodynamic disturbance is an increase in TPR. At this stage, cardiac output is low-normal to normal, and intravascular volume is contracted inversely to the increase in TPR (11). Studies during exercise show a clearly elevated TPR in these subjects and an abnormally low cardiac output due to insufficient increase in stroke volume (10). Echocardiographic studies in these subjects revealed an increase of left ventricular wall thickness, usually at the expense of chamber volume, and impaired diastolic function of the left ventricle, whereas systolic function (ejection fraction) was found to be normal (12,13).

III. HEMODYNAMIC FINDINGS IN HYPERTENSIVE WOMEN

While women were included in many of the studies of hemodynamic patterns of hypertension, it was generally assumed that the findings are identical in men and women, although it had been noted as long ago as 1913 that the prognosis of hypertension

Table 1 Selected Findings in Women and Men with Essential Hypertension Grouped According to Age

| | Patients | | | | p value | | |
| | Younger than 45 years | | Older than 45 years | | | | |
	Women	Men	Women	Men	Age	Sex	X
Age (yr)	38 ± 6	38 ± 7	56 ± 7	56 ± 7	a	a	a
Systolic pressure (mm Hg)	159 ± 16	154 ± 16	170 ± 18	172 ± 22	<0.01	NS	<0.05
Diastolic pressure (mm Hg)	91 ± 9	95 ± 10	90 ± 9	91 ± 11	NS	<0.001	NS
Cardiac output (L/min)	6.6 ± 1.3	5.9 ± 0.8	5.6 ± 1.1	5.5 ± 1.1	<0.05	<0.05	NS
Cardiac index (L/min/m^2)	3.4 ± 0.6	2.9 ± 0.4	3.0 ± 0.5	2.9 ± 0.6	<0.05	<0.05	NS
Stroke volume (ml/beat)	95 ± 17	86 ± 13	79 ± 17	82 ± 16	<0.05	NS	<0.05
Heart rate (beats/min)	70 ± 10	69 ± 9	72 ± 12	68 ± 11	NS	NS	NS
Total peripheral resistance index (U/m^2)	35 ± 7	39 ± 7	41 ± 7	42 ± 9	<0.05	<0.01	NS
Pulse pressure (mm Hg)	68 ± 12	59 ± 10	81 ± 14	81 ± 19	<0.001	<0.05	<0.05
Total blood volume (ml)	4557 ± 752	5136 ± 706	4190 ± 604	4683 ± 615	<0.05	<0.001	NS
Red cell mass (ml)	1591 ± 280	2076 ± 384	1462 ± 238	1791 ± 372	<0.05	<0.001	NS
Plasma volume (ml)	2966 ± 537	3059 ± 451	2728 ± 388	2892 ± 404	NS	NS	NS

All data are expressed as mean ± SD.
NS = not significant.
[a] p values are equal by design of the study.
Source: Ref. 15.

is better for women than men (14). However, a study from our institution demonstrated that systemic hemodynamic values and intravascular volumes differ between men and women with essential hypertension (15). When compared to men who had the same degree of blood-pressure elevation, women had a higher systemic blood flow, heart rate, and pulse pressure; a lower TPR; and a slightly more contracted intravascular volume. In addition, the blood-pressure response to isometric exercise was significantly lower. Interestingly, when men and women were grouped according to age, these differences in cardiovascular pathophysiology were more pronounced in younger patients and did not occur after age 45 (Table 1). Thus, the higher cardiac output and lower peripheral resistance found in women matched for age and arterial pressure with men resemble a hemodynamic pattern associated with the earlier stages of hypertension; that is, they are hemodynamically younger than men of the same chronological age. However, this "juvenile" hemodynamic pattern in women seems to last only until menopause; thereafter the pattern is not significantly different from that seen in men. These findings point to the sex hormones as the potential cause for these differences. While reports on the effects of estrogens used in oral contraceptives on arterial pressure are contradictory—some suggest a small increase (16,17), others report a decrease in arterial pressure (18,19)—oral contraceptives have been shown to increase cardiac output, with a proportional decrease in TPR in healthy young women (20). In addition, a recent study demonstrated that pretreatment of rat thoracic aortic rings with β-estradiol attenuates their contractile response to both phenylephrine and angiotensin II (21), indicating that that β-estradiol may have a general inhibitory effect on vascular smooth muscle function.

IV. CARDIAC ADAPTATION TO HYPERTENSION

The most important cardiac adaptation to essential hypertension is left ventricular hypertrophy (LVH) (13). While this was long thought to be a useful adaptive process allowing myocardial stress to remain normal despite an increased hemodynamic burden, data from the Framingham cohort demonstrated that LVH, determined by either electrocardiography or echocardiography, is a powerful independent risk factor for myocardial infarction, sudden death, congestive heart failure, and other cardiovascular morbidity and mortality (22,23).

Numerous studies have indicated that, in addition to arterial pressure, other factors such as age, race, body weight, and sex greatly influence left ventricular mass in both normotensives and hypertensives (24). Most studies demonstrated that the prevalence of LVH by echocardiographic criteria is consistently lower in women than in men, independent of the level of blood pressure (25–27). A study from our institution investigated left ventricular structural and functional adaptation to mild essential hypertension in a population of premenopausal and postmenopausal women who were carefully matched with the same number of men with regard to mean arterial pressure, age, and race (28). Our findings demonstrated a thinner posterior wall, a smaller left ventricular systolic and diastolic diameter, and a smaller left ventricular mass in women compared with men, even when indexed for body surface area (Table 2). In addition, indices of left ventricular performance, such as ejection fraction, velocity of circumferential fiber shortening, and a load-independent contractility index, were higher in women than men (Table 3).

However, these differences in left ventricular structure and function between women and men were more pronounced in premenopausal women and tended to disappear after the menopause. Confirming our results, an age-related increase in left ventricular mass was recently reported for women but not for men from a cross-sectional study in the normal population (29) (Figure 2). As with the disparate findings in systemic hemodynamics, the differences in cardiac adaptation between the two sexes seem to reflect the effects of the female and male hormones on the cardiovascular system. While endogenous androgens exert a trophic effect on cardiac muscle, thereby rendering men more susceptible to the deleterious effects of increased left ven-

Table 2 Echocardiographic Indexes of Left Ventricular Dimensions

	Premenopausal women (n = 15)	Men (n = 15)	Postmenopausal women (n = 14)	Men (n = 14)
End-disastolic posterior wall thickness (mm)	8.8 ± 1.2	10.1 ± 1.2[a]	9.5 ± 1.9	10.2 ± 1.5
End-diastolic septal wall thickness (mm)	10.2 ± 1.3	10.6 ± 1.4	10.2 ± 1.4	10.8 ± 1.3
End-diastolic diameter (mm)	46.3 ± 4.5	49.8 ± 4.6[a]	46.6 ± 5.4	49.9 ± 5.1
End-systolic diameter (mm)	27.6 ± 3.5	33.7 ± 4.5[b]	29.3 ± 4.8	3.35 ± 4.2
End-systolic posterior wall thickness (mm)	15.0 ± 1.7	16.1 ± 2.3	16.9 ± 2.6	16.6 ± 1.9
Left ventricular mass (g)	177 ± 46	218 ± 35[c]	192 ± 63	229 ± 48
Left ventricular mass index (g/m^2)	98 ± 21	110 ± 17	105 ± 29	112 ± 20

Values are mean ± standard deviation of the mean.
[a]$p < 0.05$.
[b]$p < 0.001$.
[c]$p < 0.02$.
Source: Ref. 28.

Table 3 Echocardiographic Indices of Left Ventricular Performance

	Premenopausal women (n = 15)	Men (n = 15)	Postmenopausal women (n = 14)	Men (n = 14)
End-diastolic volume index (ml/m²)	57 ± 12	59 ± 14	56 ± 15	58 ± 12
End-systolic wall stress (10³ dynes/cm²)	46 ± 11	53 ± 11[a]	45 ± 8	55 ± 11[b]
Ejection fraction (%)	71 ± 6	60 ± 8[c]	66 ± 10	65 ± 5
Velocity of circumferential fraction shortening (cir/s)	1.49 ± 0.28	1.20 ± 0.24[d]	1.22 ± 0.28	1.12 ± 0.18
Fractional fibre shortening (%)	41 ± 5	32 ± 6[c]	36 ± 7	33 ± 4
End systolic wall stress				
End-systolic volume index (10³ dynes/cm²/ml m²)	2.97 ± 0.52	2.32 ± 0.5[d]	2.68 ± 0.75	2.55 ± 0.55

Values are mean ± standard deviation of the mean.

[a] $p < 0.05$.
[b] $p < 0.02$.
[c] $p < 0.001$.
[d] $p < 0.01$.
Source: Ref. 28.

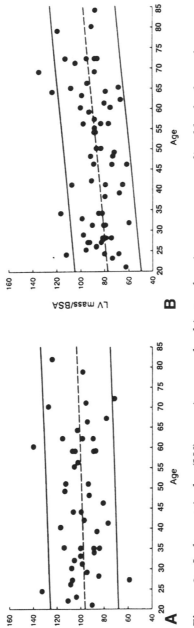

Figure 2 Left ventricular (LV) mass in normal subjects of various ages, normalized by body surface area (BSA). (A) men, (B) women. Solid lines = 95% confidence limits; dashed lines = mean values. (From Ref. 29.)

tricular mass, estrogen or its derivatives may exert some positive inotropic effect on the myocardium of premenopausal women, giving rise to an enhanced left ventricular performance. Both the different systemic hemodynamic findings and the altered cardiac adaptation to essential hypertension may be a major pathogenetic mechanism accounting for the lower risk of congestive heart failure and other cardiovascular morbidity and mortality in premenopausal women when compared to postmenopausal women or to men.

V. PATHOGENESIS OF HYPERTENSION

It is generally held that the pathogenesis of hypertension is not different in men and women, exept for the forms related to pregnancy and oral contraceptives. While the basic underlying cause of hypertension remains obscure, a large volume of research into both the pathophysiology and epidemiology of hypertension has identified certain areas, discussed below, that at least participate in the development of a persistently elevated vascular resistance, the hemodynamic hallmark of primary hypertension.

A. Activity of the Sympathetic Nervous System

Overactivity of the sympathetic nervous system, either through increased exposure or sensitivity to stress or genetically determined, has long been suspected to play an important role in the development and maintenance of primary hypertension. Support for this hypothesis comes from a variety of different investigations, i.e., the demonstration that the elevated cardiac output in the early stages of hypertension is most likely due to increased sympathetic stimulation of the heart (30). While many of these investigations include invasive procedures, such as the placement of an arterial line, there was some concern that the increased sympathetic drive reflected the emotional reaction to these procedures; however, similar findings have been reported in noninvasive studies (31). Further evidence that the sympathetic nervous system has a major role in the etiology of hypertension comes from studies in normotensive offspring of hypertensive parents, demonstrating increased plasma norepinephrine levels and total increased norepinephrine spillover (32), increased plasma norepinephrine response to mental stress (33), and increased sensitivity of isolated resistance vessels to norepinephrine (34).

In addition, there is ample evidence that people exposed to high levels of stress will develop hypertension more frequently (35,36). In turn, people in a "low-stress" environment, such as nuns and certain populations in rural, protected societies, are known to have low blood pressures that do not increase with advancing age (37,38). However, Poulter et al. (38) demonstrated that when members of these low-blood-pressure populations migrate to urban settings, they will develop higher blood pressures and a rise with advancing age.

In recent years, another approach for the assessment of sympathetic tone—power spectral analysis of heart rate and blood-pressure variability—has become increasingly popular. By computer analysis of the small, spontaneous, beat-by-beat oscillations of heart rate and systolic blood pressure, a spectrum with low- and high-frequency components can be identified that can be used as a marker for sympathetic and vagal activity, respectively. When this technique was applied to patients with essential hypertension and normotensive controls, a distinctly different pattern was found in the hypertensives, suggesting sympathetic predominance of blood-pressure and heart-rate control (39). Whether there are gender differences in the importance of the sympathetic nervous system activity as a pathogenetic factor in essential hypertension is unknown. However, the finding that heart rate is higher and volume contraction is more pronounced in hypertensive premenopausal women compared with men and postmenopausal women (15) could be explained by an increased sympathetic outflow, possibly mediated by higher estrogen levels.

B. The Renin-Angiotensin System

The renin-angiotensin system (RAS) is centrally involved in blood-pressure regulation; therefore, it may play a critical role in the pathogenesis of hypertension. Of particular interest is the final product of this system, angiotensin II, a potent vasoconstrictive hormone. While studies did not find a convincing relationship between circulating hormone levels and the height of blood pressure (40), recent research demonstrated the existence of local, noncirculating renin-angiotensin systems within the brain, reproductive tract, and cardiovascular system that might play an important role in the primary clinical observation that ACE inhibitors have been shown to be effective antihypertensive agents, even when circulating renin levels are low or even practically unmeasurable, as seen in anephric patients undergoing hemodialysis (44).

The pathogenetic mechanism that might lead to activation of the RAS in primary hypertension is not yet well established, but several hypotheses have been put forward, such as nephron heterogeneity with a population of ischemic nephrons contributing excess renin (45), increased sympathetic drive (46), or defective feedback regulation of renin-angiotensin within the kidney and the adrenal glands (47).

Studies in animal models suggest that the responsiveness of the RAS in hypertension is modulated by female sex hormones. In salt-sensitive rats, female gender not only attenuated that severity of this form of hypertension, but also influenced the relative roles of vasopressin and the renin-angiotensin system, making the RAS a relatively more important contributor to the level of hypertension (48). In contrast, ovariectomy in spontaneously hypertensive rats reduced blood pressure, active renin, and angiotensin II immunoreactivity (49).

C. Sodium Intake

Several epidemiological studies as well as studies in animal models clearly support a role of sodium in the pathogenesis of hypertension. The largest and most complete epidemiological study to date is the Intersalt study (50), in which 24-hour urine electrolytes and arterial blood pressure were measured in 10,079 men and women, aged 20 to 59, in 52 centers in 32 countries around the world. When the data of all 52 centers were combined, a significant positive correlation between sodium excretion and blood pressure was found after adjusting for confounding variables, but the association between median sodium excretion and the slope of the regression line between pressure rise and advancing age was even more impressive, indicating the importance of sodium intake in the development of hypertension. Furthermore, studies in genetically predisposed animal models clearly demonstrated the importance of high sodium intake in the pathogenesis of hypertension (51) and hypertensive heart disease (52). The major pathogenetic mechanism may be an increase in intravascular volume accompanied by an inadequate fall in TPR. However, since almost everyone in Western countries ingests a high-sodium diet but only about 50% will eventually develop hypertension, there must be differences in the sensitivity to a high sodium load. Thus, an additional renal defect in sodium excretion has been proposed as the most likely explanation for this increased "sodium sensitivity" (53).

No studies are available that demonstrate gender differences in sodium sensitivity, but such a difference seems unlikely given the association of an inheritable renal defect with sodium sensitivity. However, it is possible that sodium-sensitive premenopausal women could have a less pronounced blood-pressure response to sodium loading due to the vasodilatory effects of estrogen. After menopause, this advantage would disappear and thus contribute to the rise in blood pressure seen in this group of women.

D. Insulin Resistance

Over the last several years, a growing body of data demonstrated a relationship of hyperinsulinemia and insulin resistance with hypertension. While this association has been known to play an important part in the pathogenesis of hypertension in the obese

(54), other studies showed a marked decrease of insulin sensitivity in up to 50% of the nonobese hypertensive patients as well (55,56). These findings are supported by prospective follow-up observations indicating an up to threefold increase in the relative risk of developing hypertension in those with elevated fasting insulin levels (57) and by the presence of insulin resistance in normotensive offspring of hypertensive parents (58). The mechanisms through which hyperinsulinemia and insulin resistance lead to elevated blood pressure are not entirely clear, but it has been shown that insulin increases renal tubular absorption of transport, possibly leading to increased intracellular calcium levels that in turn could result in an enhanced vascular response to vasopressor substances (61).

Since insulin resistance is also associated with diabetes mellitus, obesity, and lipid abnormalities (particularly increased levels of triglycerides and reduced levels of HDL-C, but also slightly increased levels of LDL-C), and may contribute to the direct pathogenesis of atherosclerosis, it could represent a key factor accounting for the clustering of these disorders and therefore be responsible for a good part of cardiovascular morbidity and mortality in these patients (54). However, not all studies showed a positive relationship of hyperinsulinemia and insulin resistance with hypertension. While markedly elevated plasma insulin levels have been found in Pima Indians, blood pressure was not significanlty correlated with the fasting insulin level or the rate of glucose disposal, and they do not have an increased incidence of hypertension (62). In addition, patients with insulinomas and therefore marked hyperinsulinemia have not been found to be hypertensive (63). The conflicting results may be partly explained by different genetic mechanisms in certain ethnic groups, the influence of environmental factors, and the assumption that insulin resistance rather than hyperinsulinemia is primarily related to hypertension (64).

Interestingly, when the association of hyperinsulinemia with cardiovascular disease risk was compared in men and women, high insulin levels appeared to be linked to cardiovascular disease in men only (65). In fact, all excess risk of cardiovascular disease in men was confined to hyperinsulinemic individuals, in whom at least one of the GOH conditions (glucose intolerance, obesity, and hypertension) was present. Conversely, insulin levels were not related to cardiovascular risk in women, except in those with hypertension and high triglyceride and low HDL-C levels. A simple explanation for these surprising findings was offered in an accompanying editorial (66): Body-fat distribution rather than insulin resistance could be the main determinant of excess cardiovascular risk in this study. Body-fat distribution is determined by sex hormones and differs in men and women. Excess body fat is associated with hyperinsulinemia and insulin resistance but is associated with increased cardiovascular risk only when the fat distribution follows a "male" pattern, that is, increased upper-body fat deposition (apple-shaped). In contrast, women typically show a gluteofemoral fat distribution (pear-shaped).

While this hypothesis is a very attractive explanation for the sex differences seen in the importance of insulin resistance as a cardiovascular risk factor, it does not explain the marked increase in cardiovascular morbidity and mortality in postmenopausal women, since body-fat distribution is not changed significantly.

VI. CONCLUSIONS

Studies in our laboratory demonstrated that hypertensive women have a hemodynamic profile different from that of their male counterparts. Premenopausal women had a higher systemic blood flow, heart rate, and pulse pressure; a lower TPR; a more contracted intravascular volume; and a lower blood-pressure response to isometric exercise when compared to men with the same blood pressure. Thus, premenopausal women were hemo-dynamically younger than men of the same chronological age, leaving women less vulnerable to the deleterious effects of hypertension. In addition, women showed a more favorable cardiac adaptation to essential hypertension with a lower left ventricular mass and better systolic function. However, these sex differences disappeared after the menopause, possibly indicating that estrogens exert a protective effect on the cardiovascular system. This view is supported by numerous studies demonstrating a direct effect of estrogen on the arterial wall, leading to attenuation of vasopressor responses and inhibition of proliferation of vascular smooth-muscle cells.

Although only little data are available evaluating sex differences of contributing factors to hypertension, such as the sympathetic nervous system, the renin-angiotensin system, salt intake, and insulin resistance, it is generally assumed that the pathogenic mechanisms responsible for hypertension are not substantially different in men and women. Nevertheless, women do show an increased incidence of hypertension after menopause along with a markedly increased cardiovascular risk, and it is not yet clear whether the missing effect of estrogens on the vasculature is the only factor responsible for this phenomenon.

REFERENCES

1. Pickering GW. High Blood Pressure. London: Churchill-Livingstone, 1995:312.
2. McKee PA, Castelli WP, McNamara PM, Kannel WB. The natural history of congestive heart failure: The Framingham Study. N Engl J Med 1971; 285:1441–1446.
3. Kannel WB, Doyle JT, Ostfeld AM, et al. Optimal resources for primary prevention of atherosclerotic diseases: Atherosclerosis Study Group. Circulation 1984; 70:157A–205A.
4. Eaker ED, Castelli WP: Coronary heart disease and its risk factors among women in the Framingham Study. In: Eaker ED, Packard B, Wenger NK, Clarkson TB, Tyroler HA, eds. Coronary Heart Disease in Women: Proceedings of an NIH Workshop. Bethesda, MD: National Heart, Lung, and Blood Institute, National Institutes of Health, 1987.
5. Kannel WB, Wilson PWF. Risk Factors that attenuate the female coronary disease advantage. Arch Intern Med 1995; 155:57–61.
6. Messerli FH, De Carvalho JGR, Christie B, Frohlich ED. Systemic and regional hemodynamics in low, normal and high cardiac output borderline hypertension. Circulation 1978; 58:441–448.

7. Ventura HO, Messerli FH, Aristimuno GG, Oigman W, Suarez DH, Dreslinski GR, Dunn FG, Reisin E, Frohlich ED. Impaired systemic arterial compliance in borderline hypertension. Am Heart J 1984; 108:132–136.
8. Fujita T, Noda H. The hemodynamics in young patients with borderline hypertension. Jpn Circ J 1983; 47:795–801.
9. Messerli FH, Ventura HO, Reisin E, Dreslinski GR, Dunn FG, MacPhee AA, Frohlich ED. Borderline hypertension and obesity: Two prehypertensive states with elevated cardiac output. Circulation 1982; 66:55–60.
10. Lund-Johansen P, Omvik P. Hemodynamic patterns of untreated hypertensive disease. In: Laragh JH, Brenner BM, eds. Hypertension: Pathophysiology, Diagnosis, and Management. Vol 1. New York: Raven Press, 1990:305–327.
11. Julius S. Transition from high cardiac output to elevated vascular resistance in hypertension. Am Heart J 1988; 116:600–606.
12. Savage DD, Drayer JIM, Henry WL, Mathews EC, Ware JH, Gardin JM. Echocardiographic assessment of cardiac anatomy and function in hypertensive subjects. Circulation 1979; 59:623–632.
13. Frohlich ED, Apstein C, Chobinian AV, Devereux RB, Dustan HP, Dzau V, Fauad-Tarazi F, et al. The heart in hypertension. N Engl J Med 1992; 327:998–1008.
14. Janeway TC. A clinical study of hypertensive cardiovascular disease. Arch Intern Med 1913; 12:755–798.
15. Messerli FH, Garavaglia GE, Schmieder RE, Sundgaard-Riise K, Nunez B, Amodeo C. Disparate cardiovascular findings in men and women with essential hypertension. Ann Intern Med 1987; 107:158–161.
16. Crane MG, Harris JJ, Winsor W III. Hypertension, oral contraceptive agents, and conjugated estrogens. Ann Intern Med 1971; 74:13–21.
17. Pfeffer RI. Estrogen use, hypertension and stroke in postmenopausal women. J Chron Dis 1978; 31:389–398.
18. Von Eiff AW, Plotz EJ, Beck KJ, Czernik A. The effect of estrogens and progestins on blood pressure regulation of normotensive women. Am J Obstet Gynecol 1971; 109:887–892
19. Jespersen CM, Arnung K, Hagen C, et al. Effects of natural oestrogen therapy on blood pressure and renin-angiotensin system in normotensive and hypertensive menopausal women. J Hypertens 1983; 1:361–364.

20. Walters WAW, Yean Leng LIM. Hemodynamic changes in women taking oral contraceptives. J Obstet Gynaecol Br Commonw 1970; 77:1007–1012.

21. Ravi J, Mantzoros CS, Prabhu AS, Ram JL, Sowers JR. In vitro relaxation of phenylephrine- and angiotensin II-contracted aortic rings by beta-estradiol. Am J Hypertens 1994; 7:1065–1069.

22. Kannel WB. Prevalence and natural history of electrocardiographic left ventricular hypertrophy. Am J Med 1983; 75(suppl 3A):4–11.

23. Levy D, Garrison RJ, Savage DD, Kannel WB, Castelli WP. Prognostic implications of echocardiographically determined left ventricular mass in the Framingham heart study. N Engl J Med 1990; 322:1561–1566.

24. Messerli FH, Aepfelbacher FC. Hypertension and left ventricular hypertrophy. Cardiol Clin North Am 1995. In press.

25. Devereux RB, Alonso DR, Lutas EM, Gottlieb GJ, Campo E, Sachs I, et al. Echocardiographic assessment of left ventricular hypertrophy: comparison to necropsy findings. Am J Cardiol 1986; 57: 450–458.

26. de Simone G, Devereux RB, Roman MJ, Ganau A, Chien S, Alderman MH, et al. Gender differences in left ventricular anatomy, blood viscosity and volume regulatory hormones in normal adults. Am J Cardiol 1991; 68:1704–1708.

27. Krumholz HM, Larson M, Levy D. Sex differences in cardiac adaptation to isolated systolic hypertension. Am J Cardiol 1993; 72: 310–313.

28. Garavaglia GE, Messerli FH, Schmieder RE, Nunez BD, Oren S. Sex differences in cardiac adaptation to essential hypertension. Eur Heart J 1989; 10:1110–1114.

29. Shub C, Klein AL, Zachariah PK, Bailey KR, Tajik AJ. Determination of left ventricular mass by echocardiography in a normal population: Effect of age and sex in addition to body size. Mayo Clin Proc 1994; 69:205–211.

30. Julius S, Schork N, Schork A. Sympathetic hyperactivity in early stages of hypertension: the Ann Arbor data set. J Cardiovasc Pharmacol 1988; 12(suppl 3):S121–S129.

31. Julius S, Krause L, Schork N, et al. Hyperkinetic borderline hypertension in Tecumseh, Michigan. J Hypertens 1991; 9:77–84.

32. Ferrier C, Cox H, Esler M. Elevated total body noradrenaline

spillover in normotensive members of hypertensive families. Clin Sci 1993; 84:225–230.

33. Lenders JW, Willemsen JJ, de Boo T, et al. Disparate effects of mental stress on plasma noradrenaline in young normotensive and hypertensive subjects. J Hypertens 1989; 7:317–323.

34. Aalkjaer C, Heagerty AM, Bailey I, et al. Studies of isolated resistance vessels from offspring of essential hypertensive patients. Hypertension 1987; 9(6 Pt 2):III 155–158.

35. Cobb S, Rose RM. Hypertension, peptic ulcer, and diabetes in air traffic controllers. JAMA 1973; 224:489–492.

36. Schnall PL, Pieper C, Schwartz JE, et al. The relationship between "job strain," workplace diastolic blood pressure, and left ventricular mass index. Results of a case-control study. JAMA 1990; 263: 1929–1935.

37. Timio M, Verdecchia P, Venanzi S, et al. Age and blood pressure changes: a 20 year follow-up in nuns in a secluded order. Hypertension 1988; 12:457–461.

38. Poulter NR, Khaw KT, Hopwood BE, et al. The Kenyan Luo migration study: observations on the initiation of a rise in blood pressure. Br Med J 1990; 300:967–972.

39. Malliani A, Pagani M, Lombardi F, et al. Spectral analysis to assess increased sympathetic tone in arterial hypertension. Hypertension 1991; 17(suppl III):III36–III42.

40. Meade TW, Imeson JD, Gordon D, Peart WS. The epidemiology of plasma renin. Clin Sci 1983; 64:273–280.

41. Bunnemann B, Fuxe K, Ganten D. The brain renin-angiotensin system: localization and clinical significance. J Cardiovasc Pharmacol 1992; 19 (suppl 6):S51–S62.

42. Samani NJ. New developments in renin and hypertension: Tissue generation of angiotension I and II change the picture. Br Med J 1991; 302:981–982.

43. Dostal DE, Baker EM. Evidence for a role of an intracardiac renin-angiotensin system in normal and failing hearts. Trends Cardiovasc Med 1993; 3:67–74.

44. Man in t'Veld AJ, Schict IM, Derkx FH, de Bruyn JHB, Schalekamp MADH. Effects of an angiotensin-converting enzyme inhibitor (captopril) on blood pressure in anephric patients. Br Med J 1980; 280:288–290.

45. Sealey JE, Blumenfeld JD, Bell GM, Pecker MS, Sommers SC,

Laragh JH. On the renal basis for essential hypertension: Nephron heterogeinity with discordant renin secretion and sodium excretion causing a hypertensive vasoconstrictive-volume relationship. J Hypertens 1988; 6:763–777.

46. Julius S. Interaction between renin and the autonomic nervous system in hypertension. Am Heart J 1988; 116 (2 pt 2):611–616.

47. Williams GH, Dluhy RG, Lifton RP, et al. Non-modulation as an intermediate phenotype in essential hypertension. Hypertension 1992; 20:788–796.

48. Crofton JT, Ota M, Share L. Role of vasopressin, renin-angiotensin system and sex in Dahl salt-sensitive hypertension. J Hypertens 1993; 11:1031–1038.

49. Bachmann J, Wagner J, Haufe C, et al. Modulation of blood pressure and the renin-angiotensin system in transgenic and spontaneously hypertensive rats after ovariectomy. J Hypertens 1993; 11(suppl 5):S226–S227.

50. The Intersalt Cooperative Research Group. Intersalt: an international study of electrolyte excretion and blood pressure: Results for 24 hour urinary sodium and potassium excretion. Br Med J 1988; 297:319–328.

51. Tobian L. Salt and hypertension. Lessons from animal models that relate to human hypertension. Hypertension 1991; 17(suppl I): I52–I58.

52. Lindpaintner K, Sen S. Role of sodium in hypertensive cardiac hypertrophy. Circ Res 1985; 57:610–617.

53. Kaplam NM. Clinical Hypertension. 6th ed. Baltimore, MD: Williams & Wilkins, 1994:47–109.

54. Modan M, Halkin H, Almog S, et al. Hyperinsulnemia: A link between hypertension and obesity and glucose intolerance. J Clin Invest 1985; 75:809–817.

55. Ferrannini E, Buzzigoli G, Bonadonna R, et al. Insulin resistance in essential hypertension. N Engl J Med 1987; 317:350–357.

56. Denker PS, Pollock VE. Fasting serum insulin levels and essential hypertension: a meta-analysis. Arch Intern Med 1992; 152:1649–1651.

57. Lissner L, Bengtsson C, Lapidus L, Kristjansson K, Wedel H. Fasting insulin in relation to subsequent blood pressure changes and hypertension in women. Hypertension 1992; 20:797–801.

58. Allemann Y, Horber FF, Colombo M, et al. Insulin sensitivity and

body fat distribution in normotensive offspring of hypertensive parents. Lancet 1993; 341:327–331.

59. DeFronzo RA. The effect of insulin on renal sodium metabolism: a review with clinical implications. Diabetologica 1981; 21:165–171.

60. Landsberg L, Krieger DR. Obesity, metabolism, and the sympathetic nervous system. Am J Hypertens 1989; 2(3 pt 2):125S–132S.

61. Resnick LM. Cellular ions in hypertension, insulin resistance, obesity, and diabetes: a unifying theme. J Am Soc Nephrol 1992; 3: S78–S85.

62. Saad MF, Lillioja S, Nyomba BL, et al. Racial differences in the relation between blood pressure and insulin resistance. N Engl J Med 1991; 324:733–739.

63. Tsutsu N. Lack of association between blood pressure and insulin in patients with insulinoma. J Hypertens 1990; 8:479–484.

64. Weidmann P, de Courten M, Bohlen L. Insulin resistance, hyperinsulinemia and hypertension. J Hypertens 1993; 11(suppl 5): S27–S38.

65. Modan M, Or J, Karasik A, et al. Hyperinsulinemia, sex, and risk of atherosclerotic cardiovascular disease. Circulation 1991; 84:1165–1175.

66. Fontbonne A. Insulin: A sex hormone for cardiovascular risk? Circulation 1991; 84:1442–1444.

5

Evaluation and Clinical Findings

Vera Bittner and Suzanne Oparil

University of Alabama at Birmingham
Birmingham, Alabama

I. INTRODUCTION

Except for the forms of hypertension unique to women and those related to pregnancy and oral contraceptive therapy, the diagnosis and treatment of hypertension do not differ between the sexes. This chapter describes a systematic approach to the patient: how to establish a diagnosis of hypertension; how to classify the severity of hypertension as proposed by the Fifth Report of the Joint National Committee on Detection, Evaluation, and Treatment of High Blood Pressure (JNC V) (1); how to exclude secondary causes of hypertension; and how to determine the extent and severity of target organ damage.

II. MEASUREMENT OF BLOOD PRESSURE

The choice of equipment and the procedures for blood pressure measurement should conform to the American Heart Association's Recommendations for Human Blood Pressure Determination by Sphygmomanometers (2) and/or the American Society of Hypertension's Recommendations for Routine Blood Pressure Measurement by Indirect Sphygmomanometry (3). Blood pressure should be taken after the patient has been seated comfortably for at least 5 minutes with her arm bared, supported, and positioned at heart level. Since nicotine and caffeine can acutely increase blood pressure, the patient should not have smoked or ingested caffeine within 30 minutes prior to measurement (1). Erroneous measurements can result when the sphygmomanometer cuff size is chosen incorrectly; falsely elevated readings can be obtained when the bladder is too short, and the error is magnified if the cuff is too narrow. For accurate measurements, the cuff should be chosen such that the bladder nearly (at least 80%) or completely encircles the arm and the cuff width should cover about two thirds of the upper arm. Constriction of the upper arm by a rolled sleeve should be avoided, as it distorts the blood-pressure measurement. Patients with an arm circumference ≥33 cm require a large adult cuff, and those with an arm circumference of ≥41 cm require a thigh cuff (4). At least two readings, 2 minutes apart, should be taken at each visit and averaged. Mercury manometers are preferred, but aneroid manometers can be used, if they are standardized frequently against a mercury manometer (4). Phase I of the Korotkoff sounds is defined as the systolic blood pressure and Phase V as the diastolic blood pressure. Phase IV is used in adults only when phase V is absent (4).

III. DIAGNOSIS AND CLASSIFICATION OF HYPERTENSION

The current classification system of blood-pressure levels for adults 18 years and older, as recommended by JNC V (1), is detailed in Table 1. This classification scheme applies only to adults who are not taking antihypertensive drugs and are not acutely ill. When systolic and diastolic pressures fall into different categories, the higher category should be selected to classify the individual's blood-pressure status. Optimal blood pressure with respect to cardiovascular risk is a systolic blood pressure <120 mm Hg and a diastolic blood pressure <80 mm Hg. Unusually low readings should be evaluated for clinical significance. In addition to classifying stages of hypertension, the clinician should specify the presence or absence of target organ damage and additional risk factors to improve risk stratification and to optimize management. Pseudohypertension is occasionally present in older patients whose arteries are so rigid that they cannot be compressed by the sphygmomanometer cuff. Pseudohypertension should be suspected if there is lack of target organ damage despite consistently high blood-pressure readings and is confirmed when the pulseless radial artery remains palpable while the blood-pressure cuff is inflated to a level sufficient to obliterate the brachial pulse (Osler's sign) (5).

The diagnosis of hypertension in adults (diastolic blood pressure ≥90 mm Hg and/or systolic blood pressure ≥140 mm Hg) is made when an initial elevated reading is confirmed on at

Table 1 Classification of Blood Pressure in Adults Age 18 Years or Older

Category	Systolic (mm Hg)	Diastolic (mm Hg)
Normal	<130	<85
High normal	130–139	85–89
Hypertension		
Stage 1 (mild)	140–159	90–99
Stage 2 (moderate)	160–179	100–109
Stage 3 (severe)	180–209	110–119
Stage 4 (very severe)	≥210	≥120

Source: Ref. 1.

least two subsequent visits within one to several weeks after the initial measurement. Recommendations for follow-up based on the initial set of blood-pressure measurements are outlined in Table 2. If the systolic and diastolic categories are different, the shorter follow-up time applies. Follow-up intervals should be modified based on information about past blood-pressure measurements, other cardiovascular risk factors, or target organ disease.

Current assessments of the risk of hypertension and the benefits of treatment are based on office blood-pressure measurements. Recent data suggest, however, that damage to target organs correlates better with out-of-office measurements such as those obtained by continuous ambulatory monitoring (6–8). Although not routinely recommended, ambulatory monitoring may be useful in special clinical situations such as the evaluation of "white-coat hypertension" (which may be more common in women than in men) (9), drug resistance, nocturnal blood-pressure changes, episodic hypertension, hypotensive symptoms associated with antihypertensive medications or autonomic dysfunction, and, when performed in association with electrocar-

Table 2 Recommendations for Follow-Up Based on Initial Blood-Pressure Values

Initial screening blood pressure (mm Hg)		Recommended follow-up
Systolic	Diastolic	
<130	<85	Recheck in 2 years
130–139	85–89	Recheck in 1 year; consider advice about lifestyle modifications
140–159	90–99	Confirm within 2 months
160–179	100–109	Evaluate within 1 month
180–209	110–119	Evaluate within 1 week
≥210	≥120	Evaluate immediately

Soruce: Modified from Ref. 1.

diographic monitoring, carotid sinus syncope and pacemaker syndromes (1). The prognostic significance of white-coat hypertension remains unclear. A recent study suggests that it is associated with cardiac structural and functional changes in elderly men and women and may thus predispose to future cardiovascular events; whether treatment of such individuals would alter their natural history is unknown (10).

IV. EVALUATION OF THE PATIENT WITH NEWLY DIAGNOSED HYPERTENSION

The goals of the initial evaluation in the newly diagnosed hypertensive patient are fourfold: characterization of the patient as to age, race, lifestyle, and comorbid conditions; exclusion of secondary and thus potentially reversible causes of hypertension; identification of target organ damage; and ascertainment of other cardiovascular risk factors (1).

Essential components of the medical history and physical examination are outlined in Table 3. A detailed history of prescription and over-the-counter medication use and illicit drug use is mandatory. Drugs known to raise blood pressure or interfere with the effectiveness of antihypertensive therapy include steroids, nonsteroidal anti-inflammatory drugs, nasal decongestants, and other remedies for upper-respiratory-tract infections, appetite suppressants, cyclosporine, eythropoietin, tricyclic antidepressants, monoamine oxidase inhibitors, cocaine, and amphetamines. Recent data from the Postmenopausal Estrogen Progestin Investigation (PEPI) study suggest that hormone-replacement therapy after menopause (estrogen-only therapy or combination therapy with estrogen and a progestin) does not significantly increase blood pressure in postmenopausal women (11).

The initial laboratory evaluation consists of a urinalysis to exclude proteinuria and hematuria indicative of renal disease, creatinine to assess renal function, a complete blood count, fasting glucose, potassium level to screen for primary aldosteronism,

Table 3   Components of Patient Evaluation for Hypertension

Medical history
> Family history of high blood pressure, diabetes mellitus, dyslipidemia, and premature cardiovascular disease
> Reproductive history
> Patient history or symptoms of cardiovascular, cerebrovascular, or renal disease; diabetes mellitus; dyslipidemia; or gout.
> Known duration and levels of elevated blood pressure
> History of weight gain, leisure-time physical activities, sodium intake, and smoking and alcohol use
> Results and side effects of previous antihypertensive therapy
> Symptoms suggesting secondary hypertension
> Psychosocial and environmental factors (e.g., family situation, employment status and working conditions, educational level) that may influence blood-pressure control
> Use of medications that either raise blood pressure or interfere with the effectiveness of antihypertensive drugs

Physical examination
> Two or more blood-pressure measurements separated by 2 minutes with the patient either supine or seated, and after standing for at least 2 minutes
> Verification in the contralateral arm (if values are different, the higher value should be used)
> Measurement of height and weight

Funduscopic examination (with pupil dilatation if necessary) for arteriolar narrowing, arteriovenous compression, hemorrhages, exudates, and papilledema
> Examination of the neck for carotid bruits, distended veins, and an enlarged thyroid gland
> Examination of the heart for increased rate, increased size, precordial heave, clicks, murmurs, arrhythmias, and third (S_3) and fourth (S_4) heart sounds
> Examination of the abdomen for bruits, enlarged kidneys, masses, and abnormal aortic pulsation
> Examination of the extremities for diminished or absent peripheral arterial pulsations, bruits, and edema
> Neurological assessment

Source: Modified from Ref. 1.

calcium level to screen for hyperparathyroidism, a uric acid level, and a fasting lipid profile (total and high-density lipoprotein cholesterol and triglyceride levels). These laboratory determinations not only are useful diagnostically and for risk stratification, but also will serve as baseline measurements for future monitoring of the effects of antihypertensive treatment. A resting 12-lead electrocardiogram should also be obtained in all patients. A chest film is useful to assess heart size and may indicate underlying aortic coarctation (which should, however, be exceedingly rare as a new diagnosis among older patients). In selected individuals, ambulatory blood-pressure monitoring (see above), urinary microalbumin determination, echocardiographic assessment of cardiac anatomy and function, and plasma renin/urinary sodium determinations may be useful. If the preliminary tests show evidence of target organ damage such as retinopathy or impairment of the central nervous system, heart, kidney, or peripheral vascular system, a more detailed evaluation of the respective organ system is indicated. Because subclinical or clinically silent thyroid disease increases in prevalence with age, routine thyroid-function testing should also be strongly considered when evaluating women in the perimenopausal years and beyond.

V. EVALUATION FOR SECONDARY HYPERTENSION

Secondary hypertension other than that related to medication use is rare (<5%) in the adult hypertensive population of the United States, and routine use of elaborate and expensive diagnostic studies should be discouraged. A more detailed search for potentially reversible causes of hypertension is warranted in patients whose age, history, physical examination, severity of hypertension, or initial laboratory findings suggest secondary hypertension; in those whose blood pressure is responding poorly to therapy; in patients with well-controlled hypertension whose blood pressures begin to increase; in individuals with accelerated or malignant hypertension; and in patients with sudden onset of hypertension (often indicative of occlusive athero-sclerotic vascular disease, especially among older individuals) (1). Physical findings suggestive of secondary hypertension include abdominal or flank masses (polycystic kidney disease), abdominal bruits with a diastolic component or clear lateralization (renovascular disease), delayed or decreased lower-extremity pulses (aortic coarctation), truncal obesity with purple striae (Cushing's syndrome), tachycardia, tremor, orthostatic hypotension, sweating and pallor in the presence or absence of neurofibromas (pheochromocytoma), and muscle weakness or cramps (primary aldosteronism) (1,12).

Less than 1% of the general population of hypertensives has renovascular disease, but the prevalence may be as high as 40% among patients referred to hypertension clinics (13). Sensitivity and specificity of screening tests for renovascular hypertension are detailed in Table 4. Renal angiography with renal-vein renin measurements remains the gold standard in the diagnosis of renovascular disease, with a stenosis of >50% considered significant (13). An increased ratio of venous to arterial renin on the affected side predicts good outcome with percutaneous or surgical revascularization (13), but angioplasty is increasingly per-

Table 4 Sensitivity and Specificity of Screening Tests for Renovascular Hypertension

Test	Sensitivity (%)	Specificity (%)
Intravenous pyelogram	Approx. 75	Approx. 85
Routine renogram	80–85	75–85
Captopril renogram	93	95
Plasma renin activity (PRA)	50–80	Approx. 84
Captopril-stimulated PRA	74	89
Intravenous digital subtraction angiography	88	90
Doppler flow	84	97

Source: Ref. 14. Reproduced with permission. Copyright 1993 American Heart Association.

formed at the same time as the diagnostic angiography and without renal-vein sampling (14).

In patients with suspected hypercortisolism due to Cushing's syndrome, a 24-hour urinary-free cortisol is considered the best available test (15). The sensitivity of the test is nearly 100%, unless urine collection is incomplete, but false-positive results occur in other hypercortisolemic states. Measurement of a plasma ACTH level will distinguish between endogenous ACTH overproduction and autonomous cortisol secretion. Cranial computed tomography and magnetic resonance imaging are helpful in diagnosing pituitary and ectopic ACTH secretion in patients with elevated ACTH levels. Selected patients may require pharmacological manipulation of ACTH secretion for a definitive diagnosis.

Spontaneous or easily induced hypokalemia should raise the suspicion of underlying primary hyperaldosteronism (15). Measurement of plasma renin activity under conditions of sodium restriction, diuretic administration, and upright posture has limited sensitivity and specificity. Variability in aldosterone levels limits the usefulness of the ratio of plasma aldosterone to plasma renin activity. Measurement of aldosterone excretion rate after 3 days of salt loading is considered the single best test to detect primary aldosteronism. Patients whose aldosterone secretion rate remains greater than 14 μg/24 hr despite salt loading should undergo further evaluation, including abdominal CT scanning or magnetic resonance imaging and additional endocrinological testing to accurately determine the cause of the increased aldosterone production (16).

Pheochromocytoma can occur as an isolated tumor, in association with neurofibromatosis, or as part of one of the inherited multiple endocrine neoplasia syndromes (17). The diagnosis is established by documenting increased urinary excretion of fractionated catecholamines, metanephrines, or vanillyl-mandelic acid or elevated plasma catecholamine concentrations. Causes for potential interference with the biochemical diagnosis of pheochromocytoma are listed in Table 5 (18). Patients who are found to have elevated levels of urinary or plasma catecholamines should

Table 5   Biochemical Diagnosis of Pheochromocytoma: Sources of Interference

Stimulation of endogenous catecholamines
  Plasma and urine catecholamines are most sensitive, but metanephrines and vanillyl-mandelic acid (VMA) can be abnormal as well: emotional and physical stress, surgery, acute central nervous system disturbance, acute coronary ischemia, angiography, hypoglycemia, caffeine, nicotine, diazoxide, theophylline, drug withdrawal (alcohol, clonidine), vasodilator therapy (nitroglycerin, nitroprusside, calcium channel blockers administered acutely)

Exogenous catecholamines
  Nose drops, sinus and cough remedies, bronchodilators, appetite suppressants

Drugs altering catecholamine metabolism
  Reduction in plasma or urine catecholamines: alpha$_2$-agonists, chronic use of calcium channel blockers, converting enzyme inhibitors, bromocriptine
  Decreased VMA, increased catecholamines and metanephrines: methyldopa, monoamine oxidase inhibitors
  Variable changes: phenothiazines, tricyclic antidepressants, L-dopa
  Increase in plasma or urine catecholamines: alpha$_2$-blockers, beta-blockers, labetalol

Specific interference
  Increased metanephrines: sotalol
  Decreased metanephrines: methylglucamine in radiographic contrast medium
  Decreased urinary catecholamines: mandelamine destroys catecholamines in bladder urine
  Decreased VMA: clofibrate
  Increased VMA: nalidixic acid, anileridine
  Labetalol: metabolites interfere with all tests

Source: Modified from Ref. 18.

then undergo appropriate imaging procedures to localize the tumor(s).

VI. SUMMARY

There are no gender differences in the diagnosis and evaluation of patients with hypertension other than those relating to hypertension in pregnancy and hypertension during oral contraceptive administration. Accurate measurement of blood pressure is the cornerstone of hypertension diagnosis and management, and forms the basis for the recently revised classification system of hypertension. Patients should be classified by blood-pressure level and further characterized as to the presence or absence of end-organ damage and concomitant risk factors. Extensive testing for secondary hypertension is warranted only in patients whose initial history, physical exam, or laboratory evaluation raises the suspicion of potentially curable underlying causes.

REFERENCES

1. The Fifth Report of the Joint National Committee on Detection, Evaluation, and Treatment of High Blood Pressure (1993). Bethesda, MD: NIH publication 93-1088. U.S. Department of Health and Human Services, Public Health Service, National Institutes of Health.
2. Frohlich ED, Grim C, Labarthe DR, Maxwell MH, Perloff D, Weidman WH. Recommendations for Human Blood Pressure Determination by Sphygmomanometers. Vol 5. Report of a special task force appointed by the Steering Committee, American Heart Association. AHA publications 70–1005 (SA). Dallas: American Heart Association, 1987:i–34.
3. American Society of Hypertension. Recommendations for routine blood pressure measurement by indirect cuff sphygmomanometry. Am J Hypertens 1992; 5:207–209.
4. Grim CM, Grim CE. Blood pressure measurement. In: Izzo JL, Black HR, eds. Hypertension Primer: The Essentials of High Blood Pressure. Dallas, TX: American Heart Association, 1993:217–220.

5. Messerli FH. Osler's maneuver, pseudohypertension, and true hypertension in the elderly. Am J Med 1986; 80:906–910.

6. Perloff D, Sokolow M, Cowan RM, Juster RP. Prognostic value of ambulatory blood pressure measurements: further analyses. J Hypertens 1989; 7(suppl 3):S3–S10.

7. Parati G, Pomidossi G, Albini F, Malaspina D, Mancia G. Relationship of 24-hour blood pressure mean and variability to severity of target-organ damage in hypertension. J Hypertens 1987; 5:93–98.

8. Pickering TG, Devereux RB. Ambulatory monitoring of blood pressure as a predictor of cardiovascular risk. Am Heart J 1987; 114:925–928.

9. Pickering TG, James GD, Boddie C, Harshfield GA, Blank S, Laragh JH. How common is white coat hypertension? JAMA 1988; 259:225–228.

10. Kuwaijima I, Suzuki Y, Fujisawa A, Kuramoto K. Is white coat hypertension innocent? Hypertension 1993; 22:826–831.

11. Writing Group for the PEPI Trial. Effects of estrogen or estrogen/progestin regimens on heart disease risk factors in postmenopausal women. The Postmenopausal Estrogen/Progestin Interventions (PEPI). JAMA 1995; 273:199–208.

12. Moser M. Initial workup of the hypertensive patient. In: Izzo JL, Black HR, eds. Hypertension Primer: The Essentials of High Blood Pressure. Dallas, TX: American Heart Association, 1993:221–223.

13. Derkx FHM, Schalekamp MADH. Renal artery stenosis and hypertension. Lancet 1994; 344:237–239.

14. Nally JV Jr. Renovascular disease: Evaluation. In: Izzo JL, Black HR, eds. Hypertension Primer: The Essentials of High Blood Pressure. Dallas, TX: American Heart Association, 1993:262–264.

15. Bravo EL. Adrenal cortex: Evaluation. In: Izzo JL, Black HR, eds. Hypertension Primer: The Essentials of High Blood Pressure. Dallas, TX: American Heart Association, 1993:271–273.

16. Young WF, Hogan MJ, Klee GG, Grant CS, van Heerden JA. Primary aldosteronism: diagnosis and treatment. Mayo Clin Proc 1990; 65:96–110.

17. Sheps SG. Pheochromocytoma: Evaluation. In: Izzo JL, Black HR, eds. Hypertension Primer: The Essentials of High Blood Pressure. Dallas, TX: American Heart Association, 1993:268–270.

18. Sheps SG, Jiang NS, Klee GG. Diagnostic evaluation of pheochromocytoma. Clin Endocrinol Metab 1988; 17:397–414.

6

Concurrent Risk Factors

Gregory Y. H. Lip, John Zarifis, and Gareth Beevers
University Department of Medicine
City Hospital
Birmingham, England

I. INTRODUCTION

The menopause—spontaneous or, above all, surgically induced—is an important cardiovascular risk factor. The influence of the natural menopause on cardiovascular risk is uncertain, although it is likely that cardiovascular risk does increase. In particular, it is well recognized that coronary heart disease (CHD) is the leading cause of death in women over age 55, being responsible for one-third of all deaths in women in the United States, and with advancing age its risk increases further (1). This is pertinent because CHD in postmenopausal women has been calculated to cost the United States health service more than CHD in men (2).

Several studies have shown an association between "castration" or precocious menopause and an increased incidence of cardiovascular disease and atherosclerosis (3–9). Despite this, some population studies have failed to show any clear increase in cardiovascular morbidity and mortality at the time of the menopause. In particular, the Nurses' Health Study reported that a natural menopause was not associated with an increased risk for CHD (8). By contrast, the incidence of cardiovascular disease, as shown in the Framingham study, was two to three times greater in naturally postmenopausal and oophrectomized women when compared with premenopausal women (5). This study also showed an increase in severity of presentation of CHD, with angina being the commonest presentation among premenopausal women and death or myocardial infarction accounting for a third of CHD following the menopause (5).

Why does the menopause increase the risk of CHD? The menopause may be associated with a greater interaction between the many risk factors for cardiovascular disease. Although there is some evidence that lipid abnormalities are more common in menopausal women, there have been less consistent associations reported between the menopause and blood pressure, plasma triglycerides, glycemia, or obesity. The increased cardiovascular risk at the menopause is important because women appear significantly disadvantaged when compared to men. For example, women have a worse prognosis after a myocardial infarction or coronary artery bypass surgery (1,10–12). Female patients also have a higher operative mortality and a lower long-term bypass graft patency rate (1,11,12). In addition, proportionally fewer women receive thrombolytic therapy or are adequately investigated for coronary heart disease (1,13).

II. LIPIDS

The main difference in cardiovascular risk between men and premenopausal women has been explained by the "lipid hypothesis," which is related to changes in the androgen–estrogen ratio at the menopause. In general, androgens lower plasma high-density lipoprotein (HDL) cholesterol and increase low-density lipoprotein (LDL) cholesterol, while estrogens have the opposite effect. In healthy women, the menopause results in a loss of the protective effect of estrogens, causing a change toward a more atherogenic lipoprotein pattern, with a decline in HDL and a rise in total and LDL cholesterol. This change is also associated with a rise in heart disease to levels equal to those in men.

The increase in serum cholesterol levels after the menopause is well established, and has been reported in many studies from America (14–18), Japan (19,20), and Sweden (21). Furthermore, two longitudinal studies have also shown a rise in serum cholesterol levels (15,21). However, no difference in total cholesterol between pre- and postmenopausal women has been reported in American (Pima) Indian women (22) and American black women (16).

Although the reasons for the rise in serum cholesterol at the menopause are unclear, it is probably related to changes in lipid metabolism and hepatic processing, rather than to a change in dietary intake. In the Framingham Study, for example, there was little evidence for a relationship between total serum cholesterol and dietary fat intake (23).

However, the largest increase in total cholesterol actually occurs just before the menopause. A 10-year longitudinal study by van Beresteyn et al. (24) demonstrated that there was a mean increase of 1.08 mmol/L per 4 premenopausal years, 0.6 mmol/L per 4 early postmenopausal years, and 0.17 mmol/L during the late postmenopausal years. Similarly, Ushiroyama et al. (20) found that the rise in triglyceride and LDL cholesterol was most marked just before the onset of the menopause, suggesting a relationship with the decline of estrogen levels.

Other changes in lipid components also occur. For example, apolipoprotein A1, apolipoprotein B, triglycerides, and lipoprotein (a) are significantly higher in postmenopausal compared with premenopausal women (17,25). These effects of the menopause have been shown to be independent of age, smoking, blood pressure, and weight. Postmenopausal women also have increased levels of circulating, small, dense LDL particles, which are considered to further increase the risk for the development of atherosclerosis (26).

III. HYPERTENSION

Cross-sectional and longitudinal studies have shown a progressive rise in blood pressure with age. During the first four or five decades, the incidence of hypertension is higher in men than in women. Beyond the age of 50 years, however, the incidence of hypertension increases at a faster rate in women (27). The increase in blood pressure with age is influenced by racial origin, with black or Afro-Caribbean hypertensives having a greater increase than white patients (28).

The menopause itself is accompanied by a rise in systolic and diastolic blood pressures—independent of age—resulting in a higher prevalence of hypertension in women who are postmenopausal compared with those in the premenopausal state (29). Some workers have suggested that the blood-pressure rise with increasing age may be related to the decrease in production of endogeneous female hormone that accompanies the menopause (30). An increase in body weight is also an important and potentially preventable determinant of the increased blood pressure and prevalence of hypertension in postmenopausal women (31). In addition, the menopause is associated with enhanced stress-induced cardiovascular responses and elevated ambulatory blood pressures during the workday (32).

Hypertension is an important cardiovascular risk factor. For example, CAD is twice as common in hypertensive patients as in the normotensive population (33,34). Pooled clinical trial results have demonstrated that a reduction in diastolic blood pressure by 5–6 mm Hg results in a 35–40% reduction in stroke and a 20–25% reduction in CHD (33). The treatment of hypertension and good blood-pressure control is thus essential in postmenopausal women because a combination of cardiovascular risk factors adds to an increased cardiovascular risk "load" for individual women.

If end-organ damage is present in hypertensives, this confers additional cardiovascular risk. Examples of end-organ damage in hypertensives includes the presence of left ventricular hypertrophy (LVH) and microalbuminuria.

A. Left Ventricular Hypertrophy

Left ventricular hypertrophy is common and can be considered an adaptive state of the heart to increased ventricular wall stress in hypertension. Approximately 50% of patients with diastolic blood pressures between 110 and 120 mm Hg have ECG criteria for LVH, and the prevalence increases with age. The presence of LVH has considerable prognostic implications (34). In particular, hypertensives with LVH have an increased risk of sudden death, arrhythmias (including ventricular arrhythmias and atrial fibrillation), and hypertensive heart failure. In addition, there is a 12-fold increase in the risk of stroke, a fourfold increase in the risk of acute myocardial infarction, and a threefold increase in intermittent claudication if LVH is present (34). After adjusting for confounding factors, the relative risk of a coronary event in men and women increased by 1.67 and 1.60, respectively, for every 50 g/m increment in left ventricular mass per unit of height (35).

Heart failure in hypertensives with LVH can functionally be related to both systolic and diastolic dysfunction (34). In particular, left ventricular systolic function is reduced in about 15% of hypertensive patients (which may be related to an increased risk of cardiac ischaemia, myocardial infarction, and arrhythmias). However, heart failure in hypertensives can occasionally be due to diastolic dysfunction, with a poorly relaxing, noncompliant left ventricle, that results in pulmonary congestion (36).

B. Microalbuminuria

Low-level (20–200 mg/24 hour) albuminuria ("microalbuminuria") is an additional independent predictor of cardiovascular risk at all ages, the excretion rate increasing with age in men but not women (37). Microalbuminuria has been correlated with raised blood pressure in hypertensive patients, and is predictive of morbidity and mortality from cardiovascular disease (38,39). This association has two possible explanations (38): microalbuminuria is associated with an excess of known cardiovascular risk factors (such as lipid abnormalities and diabetes); in addition, it may be a marker of established cardiovascular disease.

In hypertension, microalbuminuria has been correlated with abnormal plasma levels of von Willebrand factor, an index of endothelial dysfunction (39). This suggests that albuminuria in essential hypertension may reflect systemic dysfunction of the vascular endothelium, and this in turn contributes to increased vascular risk. In addition, patients with essential hypertension and microproteinuria have higher blood pressures and a higher prevalence of echocardiographic and electrocardiographic LVH (40).

IV. OBESITY AND BODY MASS INDEX

Being overweight is a risk factor, and cardiovascular risk is generally associated with central obesity and a high waist-to-hip ratio (41–43). However, the precise role of obesity as an independent cardiac risk factor remains unclear.

The contribution of weight gain, obesity, and body mass index to cardiovascular risk after the menopause remains uncertain. Postmenopausal women have a greater (20%) fat mass and a higher proportion of android (upper-body) fat when compared to premenopausal women (43,44). There is also a general belief that women have a tendency to gain weight after the menopause. However, an increase in body weight is associated with the increased prevalence of hypertension in postmenopausal women (31). Although analysis of the Framingham data demonstrates an independent contribution to the risk of coronary disease by hypertension, and high levels of serum cholesterol, glucose, and urate, these factors are all increased with an increasing body mass index (45).

Weight gain at the time of the menopause, and the effects on coronary heart disease risk factors, was prospectively studied by Wing et al. (43) in a population-based sample of 485 women.

They found no significant differences in weight gain (approximately 20% gained 4.5 kg or more) over the 3-year follow-up between postmenopausal women and those who remained premenopausal (43). However, weight gain was significantly associated with increases in blood pressure and levels of total cholesterol, LDL cholesterol, triglycerides, and fasting insulin levels (43). A rise in weight at the menopause may thus explain some of the changes in coronary heart disease risk factors (45).

In epidemiological studies, however, relative body weight does not appear to have a consistent relationship to a natural menopause. For example, the menopause has been shown to affect blood pressure and weight gain in studies from the United states Health Examination Survey (14) and Scandinavia (21, 46,47). By contrast, no relationship was seen in the Framingham Study (15) and from studies in Japan (48). Lindquist (21) suggests that a gain in weight with time is seen in recently postmenopausal women, but, in the long run, it is likely that the menopause actually results in weight loss.

V. PHYSICAL ACTIVITY

The role of physical activity as a preventive measure against CHD and in decreasing mortality after myocardial infarction remains controversial. An exercise program for menopausal women is usually advocated as having beneficial effects in the prevention of cardiovascular disease, obesity, and osteoporosis. Long-term physical activity is important in maintaining an ideal body weight postmenopause, and exercise may also play a role in maintaining normal blood pressure and optimizing lipid values.

Decreased levels of physical fitness are associated with an increased risk of atherosclerosis (49). The relative risk for cardiovascular disease conferred by physical inactivity appears to be similar in magnitude to the risk conferred by hypertension, lipid abnormalities, or smoking (50). In addition to a role as a primary risk factor for the development of CHD, physical inactivity may also affect the secondary association of other cardiac risk factors.

For example, the Framingham Offspring Study reported that subjects who exercised for at least 1 hour weekly had an improved cardiac risk profile when HDL cholesterol, heart rate, body mass index, and smoking were analyzed (51).

VI. PROTHROMBOTIC FACTORS AND ABNORMALITIES IN ENDOTHELIAL FUNCTION

Plasma fibrinogen is well established as another cardiovascular risk factor, and high levels of plasma fibrinogen levels are associated with cardiovascular disease and stroke (52,53). Abnormalities in hemostatic function favoring thrombosis may promote a prothrombotic or hypercoagulable state and will have important prognostic implications, especially if concomitant vascular disease is already present (54). Other markers, such as plasma von Willebrand factor (vWF), may be related to abnormal endothelial function, thus promoting thrombogenesis and atherogenesis (55). Elevated levels of plasma vWF have, for example, been found in hypertensives (39,55,56) and in patients with CHD (57,58); in the latter group, high vWF levels are predictive of recurrent myocardial infarction (57). Abnormalities in prothrombotic factors and endothelial dysfunction may therefore account in part for the increased risk for ChD at the time of the menopause, and have important prognostic implications.

There is usually a postmenopausal rise in plasma fibrinogen, factor VII, and other prothrombotic factors (59–64). The Northwick Park Heart Study showed, for example, that mean levels of factor VIIc, fibrinogen, and cholesterol were between 6 and 10% higher in postmenopausal women than in premenopausal women (61). This would be equivalent to an increase in the risk of fatal ischemic heart disease in postmenopausal women by about 40% compared with premenopausal women of the same age (61). Premenopausal women had lower plasma levels of fibrinogen, factor VIIc, and antithrombin III compared to postmenopausal women (60).

Concomitant cardiovascular risk factors discussed above may have an important interaction with prothrombotic factors. For example, smoking is strongly associated with high fibrinogen levels (52,53). In obese patients (body mass index >30), plasma viscosity and fibrinogen levels are also significantly higher than those in healthy, nonobese subjects (body mass index <25) (65,66). This difference is independent of the presence of atherosclerotic complications and other risk factors.

Strenuous exercise is associated with lower plasma fibrinogen (and cholesterol) concentrations, which is equivalent to a difference of 15% in the risk of ischemic heart disease, when compared to a sedentary lifestyle (67). Similar changes of plasma fibrinogen with exercise were seen in the Caerphilly Prospective Heart Study, the Scottish Health Heart Study, and the Gothenburg study (63,65,68). As discussed below, postmenopausal treatment with hormone replacement therapy has important beneficial effects on these prothrombotic factors.

VII. INSULIN RESISTANCE AND DIABETES

Diabetes seems to have greater impact in women, with regard both to the incidence of CHD and to prognosis. The incidence of coexistent hypertension and diabetes is greater than would be expected if they were considered separately (69–73). However, hypertension in diabetics (especially those with non-insulin-dependent diabetes mellitus) occurs more often in women over 50 years old than in men (69,70). It is not clear whether the risk of vascular disease in hypertensive diabetics is independent of the upper-body obesity, lower HDL cholesterol levels, and higher triglyceride levels seen in women with diabetes. Triglycerides are also said to contribute to the risk of heart disease particularly in diabetic women (74). However, lipoprotein (a) does not appear to contribute to the difference in the prevalence of CAD between diabetics and nondiabetics (75).

The fasting insulin level is increasingly being cited as a cardiovascular risk factor (76,77). High insulin levels in the presence of normal or slightly elevated blood glucose levels are suggestive of underlying insulin resistance. Even in nondiabetics, there is a strong association among plasma glucose, insulin levels, insulin resistance, and the risk of CHD (76,77). Two possible mechanisms (77,78) can explain this. First, a primary defect of insulin resistance may occur, and the associated high insulin levels are causally related to some cardiovascular risk factors—independently or in combination—leading to the development of atherosclerotic vascular disease. Alternatively, the insulin resistance may indicate a cellular defect that is related to both cardiovascular risk factors and atherosclerosis.

However, population studies have reported that natural menopause does not alter glucose tolerance and insulin levels, in the absence of other predisposing factors such as obesity and a history of gestational or familial diabetes mellitus (15,79,80). In contrast, a recent report suggests that healthy postmenopausal women subjected to an insulin-tolerance test will demonstrate a high prevalence of insulin resistance, and that estrogen use increases, while progestins decrease, insulin sensitivity (80).

The beneficial effect of hormone replacement therapy (HRT) may also be due in part to some alterations in these metabolic factors. For example, lower levels of fasting glucose and insulin have also been found in women taking both estrogen-only and combined HRT preparations (81,82).

VIII. SMOKING

Smoking is recognized as a major risk factor for CHD (83–87). Although the overall incidence of smoking is decreasing in the Western world, there are now more women smoking (85–87). Women who avoid or stop smoking are generally those who are better educated and more enlightened, and are already at a lower risk of CHD. Furthermore, women find it more difficult than men to give up smoking, perhaps partly because of a fear of gaining weight. The role of smoking as a risk factor is particularly important because the risk of developing CHD is higher in female smokers than in male smokers (87).

In addition, smoking increases the risk of early menopause (88). A study by Schlemmer et al. (89) suggests that smoking may induce an increase in androgen levels in early postmenopausal women, with higher levels of androstenedione and luteinizing hormone in smokers when compared with nonsmokers. Although smoking does not appear to be related to estradiol levels in postmenopausal women, levels of adrenal androgens are significantly increased (90).

Smoking also interacts very strongly with other important risk factors such as hyperlipidemia, prothrombotic factors, and hypertension (91), and the combined cardiovascular risk "load" will be of particular importance in the postmenopausal state. Elevated thromboxane A_2 levels are also found in women who smoke cigarettes, consistent with an increase in platelet activity that is dependent on smoking intensity (92).

IX. HORMONE REPLACEMENT THERAPY AND CONCOMITANT RISK FACTORS

Several studies have suggested a significant reduction in cardiovascular risk in postmenopausal women taking estrogen as hormone replacement therapy (93,94). In particular, there is a reduction in cardiovascular morbidity by about 35%, although the benefits in stroke reduction remain uncertain (93–96). In view of the perceived benefits of HRT in cardiovascular prevention, a recent policy statement by the American College of Physicians suggested that preventive hormone replacement therapy should be considered in all postmenopausal women (97). Despite this, there continues to be concern among general practitioners and clinicians that HRT use may result in an increased risk of venous thrombosis, stroke, myocardial infarction, and hypertension (98). Women's attitudes are also important (99,100), especially with some doubts as to whether the reported efficacy of HRT is due to a "healthy cohort" effect (101). However, HRT use may have additional benefits in the modification of risk factors associated with an increased cardiovascular risk at the menopause.

A. Hypertension

Reluctance and confusion still exist with respect to prescribing HRT to postmenopausal women who also have hypertension; many clinicians avoid its use, especially if blood pressure remains difficult to control (98). A particular concern is that HRT use may actually increase blood pressure. In younger women, for example, the use of high-dose estrogen-containing oral contraceptives may be associated with an increase in systolic and diastolic blood pressures (102,103).

In postmenopausal women the situation is less clear. In normotensive postmenopausal women, the use of HRT does not raise blood pressure and may even lower it (30,104–109). A large retrospective study of HRT in hypoestrogenic normotensive women also showed a significant reduction in the new development of hypertension in patients treated with estrogen (110).

The effects of HRT in hypertensive postmenopausal women have been less investigated, with only three studies addressing this issue in the literature. Pfeffer et al. (107) retrospectively studied 35 women (aged 52–87) with documented hypertension, in whom a fall in systolic blood pressure was demonstrated following oral estrogen therapy. In a small Danish study (111), 12 normotensive and 12 hypertensive women were prospectively started on HRT, with a fall in systolic blood pressure being demonstrated in the hypertensive group after 6 months. In an open prospective study of 75 hypertensive menopausal women, Lip et al. (112) found no change in mean blood pressure over a median follow-up of 18 months, despite a rise in mean weight. In women with uncontrolled hypertension, in whom HRT was prospectively discontinued, the same investigators found no significant fall in mean blood pressure, suggesting the lack of a significant pressor effect of HRT on blood pressure (113).

The evidence therefore suggests that HRT can safely be prescribed to hypertensive women, with additional advantages with respect to cardiovascular risk. Only a large, prospective, randomized, placebo-controlled study can allay any final doubts, although whether such a study would be feasible or ethical remains debatable. To study the effects of HRT on blood pressure in 100 symptomatic *hypertensive* postmenopausal women (and HRT would have to be withheld in 50% of them in a placebo-controlled study), it would be necessary to screen about 1000 symptomatic postmenopausal women (and therefore even more postmenopausal women to find those who are actually symptomatic) (96).

B. Lipids and Prothrombotic Factors

The use of exogenous female hormone in premenopausal women adversely affects the lipid profile and may account in part for the increased risks of cardiovascular disease in association with oral contraceptives (114–117). Postmenopausal HRT, by contrast, appears to result in beneficial alterations in the lipid profile, such as an increase in HDL cholesterol and a decrease in LDL cholesterol (105,118–121).

The effects of estrogens in HRT on blood lipids (and hemostatic factors) are thought to be antagonized by the coadministration of progestagens (especially those with androgenic properties). For example, adverse changes in lipoproteins may be induced with the use of progestagens (122–124). In the Framingham Offspring Study, estrogen use was inversely associated with LDL cholesterol and apolipoprotein B levels, while increasing progesterone content in HRT was inversely related to HDL cholesterol and apolipoprotein A-1 levels (116).

These concerns were further examined in the large Atherosclerosis Risk in Communities Study, which found that HRT users had higher HDL and lower LDL cholesterol, apolipoprotein B, lipoprotein (a), fibrinogen, antithrombin III, and fasting blood glucose and insulin levels. However, in contrast to previous studies, users of combined estrogen/progesterone HRT preparations had a better lipid and hemostatic factor profile compared to users of estrogen alone (81). The Framingham Offspring Study also showed that the use of medroxyprogesterone acetate (a progesterone with minimal androgenic properties) in combination with estrogens did not adversely affect the lipid profile (116); this improvement in lipid profile has been confirmed by others (122,125,126). The adverse effects of progesterone can therefore be minimized by using less androgenic progestagens (122). Gambrell and Teran (126) also suggest that the addition of progestogens did not adversely affect the lipid profile when adequate dosages of estrogens were used.

HRT may also improve the balance between coagulation and fibrinolysis, resulting in the reduction of a prothrombotic or hypercoagulable state. For example, women taking HRT had lower plasma fibrinogen levels and higher levels of plasma plasminogen and factor VIIc than those who were not on HRT (127).

C. Other Risk Factors

HRT has been reported to reverse the increased fat distribution that results from loss of ovarian function following the menopause, resulting in a reduction in body mass index (128). In contrast, the use of HRT in hypertensive women was associated with an increase in weight in other studies (112). It is therefore possible that HRT protects against the development of central obesity with an android distribution of body fat, with only variable effects on body mass index.

X. CONCLUSION

As the life expectancy of the population increases, a greater number of postmenopausal women would mean a higher cardiovascular disease "burden" on the population. The risks that lead to the development of cardiovascular disease are multifactorial, and hormone replacement therapy may have beneficial effects on some risk factors. Cessation of smoking, weight control, and monitoring of blood pressure and diabetes in high-risk patients are other important strategies in cardiovascular risk-factor modification in menopausal women.

ACKNOWLEDGMENTS

We thank Michèle Beevers, SRN, and David Churchill, MRCOG, for helpful advice during the preparation of this manuscript. GL is the recipient of the Edith Walsh and Ivy Powell Research Awards for cardiovascular disease from the British Medical Association.

REFERENCES

1. Eysman SB, Douglas PS. Reperfusion and revascularization strategies for coronary artery disease in women. JAMA 1992; 268: 1903–1907.
2. Vital statistics of the United States 1983. Vol II. Mortality, part B. Washington, DC: US Department of Health and Human Services Publication 87–1114, 1987.
3. Parrish HM, Carr CA, Hall DG, King TM. Time interval from castration in premenopausal women to development of excessive coronary atherosclerosis. Am J Obstet Gynecol 1967; 99:155–162.
4. Bengtsson C, Lindquist O. Coronary heart disease during the menopause. In: Oliver MF, ed. Coronary Heart Disease in Young Women. London: Churchill-Livingstone, 1978:234–239.
5. Gordon T, Kannel WB, Hjortland MC, McNamara PM. Menopause and coronary heart disease. The Framingham Study. Ann Intern Med 1978; 89:157–161.
6. Rosenberg L, Hennekens CH, Rosner B, Belanger C, Rothman KJ, Speizer FE. Early menopause and the risk of myocardial infarction. Am J Obstet Gynecol 1981; 139:47–51.
7. Svanberg L. Effects of estrogen deficiency in women castrated when young. Acta Obstet Gynecol Scand Suppl 1982; 106:11–15.
8. Colditz GA, Willett WC, Stampfer MJ, Rosner B, Speizer FE, Hennekens CH. Menopause and the risk of coronary heart disease in women. N Engl J Med 1987; 316:1105–1110.
9. Witteman JCM, Grobbee DE, Kok FJ, Hofman A, Valkenburg HA.

Increased risk of atherosclerosis in women after the menopause. Br Med J 1989; 298:642–644.

10. Lip GYH, Metcalfe MJ. Have we identified the factors affecting prognosis following coronary artery bypass surgery? Br J Clin Prac 1994; 48:317–322.

11. Findlay IN. Coronary bypass surgery in women. Curr Opin Cardiol 1994; 9:650–657.

12. Loop FD, Goldberg LR, MacMillan JP, Cosgrove DM, Lytle BW, Sheldon WC. Coronary artery surgery in women when compared with men: Analysis of risks and long-term results. J Am Coll Cardiol 1983;; 1:383–390.

13. Clarke KW. Gray D, Keating NA, Hampton JR. Do women with acute myocardial infarction receive the same treatment as men? Br Med J 1994; 309:563–566.

14. Weiss NS. Relationship of menopause to serum cholesterol and arterial blood pressure: The United States Health Examination Survey of Adults. Am J Epidemiol 1972; 96:237–241.

15. Hjortland MC, McNamara P, Kannel WB. Some atherogenic concomitants of menopause: The Framingham Study. Am J Epidemiol 1976; 103:304–311.

16. Baird DD, Tyroler HA, Heiss G, Chambless LE, Hames CG. Menopausal change in serum cholesterol: Black/White differences in Evans County, Georgia. Am J Epidemiol 1985; 122: 982–993.

17. Brown SA, Hutchinson R, Morrisett J, et al. Plasma lipid, lipoprotein cholesterol and apoprotein distributions in selected US communities: The Atherosclerosis Risk in Communities (ARIC) Study. Atheroscler Thromb 1993; 13:1139–1158.

18. Demirovic J, Sprafka JM, Folsom AR, Laitinen D, Blackburn H. Menopause and serum cholesterol: differences between blacks and whites. The Minnesota Heart Survey. Am J Epidemiol 1992; 136:155–164.

19. Shibata H, Haga H, Suyama Y, Kumagai S, Seino T. Serum total and HDL cholesterols according to reproductive status in Japanese females. J Chron Dis 1987; 40:209–213.

20. Ushiroyama T, Okamoto Y, Sugimoto O. Plasma lipid and lipoprotein levels in perimenopausal women: Clinical research in 1198 Japanese women. Acta Obstet Gynecol Scand 1993; 72: 428–433.

21. Lindquist O. Intraindividual changes of blood pressure, serum

lipids and body weight in relation to menstrual status: results from a prospective population study of women in Göteborg, Sweden. Prev Med 1982; 11L:162–172.

22. Hamman RH, Bennett PH, Miller M. The effect of menopause on serum cholesterol in American (Pima) Indian women. Am J Epidemiol 1975; 102:164–169.

23. Posner BM, Cupples LA, Miller DR, Cobb JL, Lutz KJ, D'Agostino RB. Diet, menopause and serum cholesterol levels in women: the Framingham Study. Am Heart J 1993; 125:483–489.

24. van Beresteyn ECH, Korevaar JC, Huybregts PCW, Schouten EG, Burema J, Kok FJ. Perimenopausal increase in serum cholesterol: a 10-year longitudinal study. Am J Epidemiol 1993; 137:383–392.

25. Bonithon-Kopp C, Scarabin PY, Darne B, Malmejac A, Guize L. Menopause-related changes in lipoproteins and some other cardiovascular risk factors. Int J Epidemiol 1990; 19:42–48.

26. Campos H, McNamara JR, Wilson PW, et al. Differences in low density lipoprotein subfractions and apolipoproteins in premenopausal and postmenopausal women. J Clin Endocrinol Metab 1988; 67:30.

27. von Eiff AW. Blood pressure and estrogens. Front Hormone Res 1975; 3:177–184.

28. Akinkugbe OO. World epidemiology of hypertension in blacks. In: Dallas Hall W, Saunders E, Shulman NB, eds. Hypertension in Blacks: Epidemiology, Pathophysiology and Treatment. Chicago: Year Book Publishers, 1985:3–16.

29. Staessen J, Bulpitt CJ, Fagard R, Lijnen P, Amery A. The influence of menopause on blood pressure. J Hum Hypertens 1989; 3: 427–433.

30. Regensteiner JG, Hiatt WR, Byyny RL, Tickett CK, Woodard WD, Moore LG. Short-term effects of estrogen and progestin on blood pressure of normotensive postmenopausal women. J Clin Pharmacol 1991; 31:543–548.

31. Grobbee DE, van Hemert AM, Vandenbroucke JP, Hofman A, Valkenburg HA. Importance of body weight in determining rise and level of blood pressure in postmenopausal women. J Hypertens 1988; 6(suppl 4):S614–616.

32. Owens JF, Stoney CM, Matthews KA. Menopausal status influences ambulatory blood pressure levels and blood pressure changes during mental stress. Circulation 1993; 88:2794–2802.

33. Collins R, MacMahon. Blood pressure, antihypertensive drug

treatment and the risks of stroke and of coronary heart disease. Br Med Bull 1994; 50:272–298.

34. Lip GYH, Gammage MD, Beevers DG. Hypertension and the heart. Br Med Bull 1994; 50:299–321.

35. Levy D, Garrison RJ, Savage DD, Kannel WB, Castell WP. Prognostic implications of echocardiographically determined left ventricular mass in the Framingham Heart Study. N Engl J Med 1990; 322:1561–1566.

36. Fouad-Tarazi FM. Left ventricular diastolic dysfunction in hypertension. Curr Opin Cardiol 1994; 9:551–560.

37. Gould MM, Mohamed-Ali V, Goubet SA, Yudkin JS, Haines AP. Microalbuminuria: associations with height and sex in nondiabetic subjects. Br Med J 1993; 306:240–242.

38. Winocour PH. Microalbuminuria. Br Med J 1992; 304:1196–1197.

39. Pedrinelli R, Giampietro O, Carmassi F, et al. Microalbuminuria and endothelial dysfunction in essential hypertension. Lancet 1994; 344:14–18.

40. Schmieder R, Grube E, Ruddel H, Schlebusch H, Schulte W. [Significance of microproteinuria for early detection of hypertension-induced end-organ damage.] Klin Wochenschr 1990; 68:256–262 (in German).

41. Wing RR, Matthews KA, Kuller LH, et al. Waist to hip ratio in middle-aged women: Association with behavioural and psychosocial factors and with changes in cardiovascular risk factors. Arterioscler Thromb 1991; 11:1250–1257.

42. Lapidus L, Bentsson C, Larsson B. Distribution of adipose tissue and body fat and risk of cardiovascular disease: A 12-year followup of participants in the population study of women in Gothenberg, Sweden. Br Med J 1984; 289:1257.

43. Wing RR, Matthews KA, Kuller LH, Meilahn EN, Plantinga PL. Weight gain at the time of menopause. Arch Intern Med 1991; 151:97–102.

44. Ley CJ, Lees B, Stevenson JC. Sex- and menopause-associated changes in body-fat distribution. Am J Clin Nutr 1992; 55:950–954.

45. Garrow JS. Is obesity an independent risk factor? In: Poulter N, Sever P, Thom S, eds. Cardiovascular Disease: Risk Factors and Intervention. Oxford: Radcliffe Press 1993:153–160.

46. Hallberg L, Svanborg A. Cholesterol, phospholipids and triglycerides in plasma in 50 year old women: Influence of meno-

pause, body-weight, skinfold thickness, weight gain and diet in a random population sample. Acta Med Scand 1967; 181:185–194.

47. Kuskowska-Wolk A, Rossner S. Prevalence of obesity in Sweden: cross-sectional study of a representative adult population. J Intern Med 1990; 227:241–246.

48. Shibata H, Matsuzaki T, Hatano S. Relationship of relevant factors of atherosclerosis to menopause in Japanese women. Am J Epidemiol 1979; 109:420–424.

49. Blair SN, Kohl HW, Pafffenberger PS, et al. Physical fitness and all-cause mortality: A prospective study of healthy men and women. JAMA 1989; 262:2395.

50. Powell KE, Thompson PD, Caspersen CJ, Kendrick JS. Physical activity and the incidence of coronary heart disease. Annu Rev Public Health 1987; 8:253.

51. Daneberg AL, Keller JB, Wilson PW, Castelli WP. Leisure time physical activity in the Framingham Offspring Study: Description, seasonal variation and risk factor correlates. Am J Epidemiol 1989; 129:76.

52. Ernst E, Resch KL. Fibrinogen as a cardiovascular risk factor: a meta-analysis and review of the literature. Ann Intern Med 1993; 118:956–963.

53. Lip GYH. Fibrinogen and cardiovascular disorders. Q J Med 1995; 88:155–165.

54. Fowkes FGR, Lowe GDO, Housley E, Rattray A, Rumley A, Elton RA, MacGregor IR, Dawes J. Cross-linked fibrin degradation products, progression of peripheral arterial disease, and risk of coronary heart disease. Lancet 1993; 342:84–86.

55. Lip GYH, Beevers DG. Abnormalities of rheology and coagulation in hypertension. J Hum Hypertens 1994; 8:693–702.

56. Blann AD, Naqvi T, Waite M, McCollum CN. Von Willebrand factor and endothelial damage in essential hypertension. J Hum Hypertens 1993; 7:107–111.

57. Jansson JH, Nilsson TK, Johnson O. von Willebrand factor in plasma: a novel risk factor for recurrent myocardial infarction and death. Br Heart J 1991; 66:351–355.

58. Lip GYH, Metcalfe MJ, Rumley A, Dunn FG, Lowe GDO. Plasma fibrinogen and fibrin D-dimer levels in left ventricular aneurysms: thrombogenesis and the effects of warfarin. Eur Heart J 1994; 15(suppl):589.

59. Brunner EJ, Marmot MG, White IR, et al. Gender and employ-

ment grade differences in blood cholesterol, apolipoproteins and haemostatic factors in the Whitehall II study. Atherosclerosis 1993; 102:195–207.

60. Meilahn EN, Kuller LH, Matthews KA, Kiss JE. Variation in plasma fibrinogen levels by menopausal status and use of hormone replacement therapy: the Healthy Women Study. In: Ernst E, Koenig W, Lowe GDO, Meade TW, eds. Fibrinogen: A "New" Cardiovascular Risk Factor. Vienna: Blackwell-MZV, 1992:338–343.

61. Meade TW, Haines AP, Imeson JD, Stirling Y, Thompson SG. Menopausal status and haemostatic variables. Lancet 1983; i: 22–24.

62. Scarabin PY, Bonithon-Kopp C, Bara L, Malmejac A, Guize L, Samama M. Factor VII activation and menopausal status. Thromb Res 1990; 57:227–234.

63. Lee AJ, Smith WC, Lowe GD, Tunstall-Pedoe H. Plasma fibrinogen and coronary risk factors: the Scottish Heart Health Study. J Clin Epidemiol 1990; 43:913–919.

64. Folsom AR, Wu KK, Davis CE, Conlan MG, Sorlie PD, Szklo M. Population correlates of plasma fibrinogen and factor VII, putative cardiovascular risk factors. Atherosclerosis 1991; 91:191–205.

65. Craveri A, Tornaghi G, Paganardi L, Ranieri R, Leonardi G, Di Bella M. [Hemorrheologic disorders in obese patients: Study of the viscosity of the blood, erythrocytes, plasma, fibrinogen and the erythrocyte filteration index.] Minerva Med 1987; 78:899–906.

66. Rosengren A, Wilhelmsen L, Welin L, Tsipogianni, Teger-Nilsson AC, Wedel H. Social influences and cardiovascular risk factors as determinants of plasma fibrinogen concentration in a general population sample of middle aged men. Br Med J 1990; 300: 634–638.

67. Connelly JB, Cooper JA, Meade TW. Strenuous exercise, plasma fibrinogen, and factor VII activity. Br Heart J 1992; 67:351–354.

68. Elwood PC, Yarnell JWG, Pickering J, Fehily AM, O'Brien JR. Exercise, fibrinogen and other factors for ischaemic heart disease. Br Heart J 1993; 69:183–187.

69. Christlieb AR, Warram JH, Krolewski AS, et al. Hypertension: the major risk factor in juvenile-onset insulin-dependent diabetics. Diabetes 1981; 30(suppl 2):90–96.

70. Klein BE, Klein R, Moss SE. Blood pressure in a population of

diabetic persons diagnosed after 30 years of age. Am J Pub Health 1984; 74:336–339.

71. Lipson LG. Special problems in treatment of hypertension in the patient with diabetes mellitus. Arch Intern Med 1984; 144:1829–1831.

72. Houston MD. Adverse effects of antihypertensive drug therapy on glucose intolerance. Cardiol Clin 1986; 4:117–135.

73. Fuller JH. Epidemiology of hypertension associated with diabetes mellitus. Hypertension 1985; 7:113–117.

74. Gotto AM. Hypertriglyceridaemia: Risks and perspectives. Am J Cardiol 1992; 70:19H–25H.

75. Farrer M, Game FL, Albers CJ, Neil HAW, Winocour PH, Laker MF, Adams PC, Alberti KGMM. Association between impaired glucose tolerance and circulating concentration of Lp(a) lipoprotein in relation to coronary heart disease. Br Med J 1993; 307: 832–836.

76. Stout RW. Insulin and atheroma. 20 year perspective. Diabetes Care 1990; 13:631–654.

77. Stout RW. Insulin resistance: A unifying hypothesis in cardiovascular disease. In: Poulter N, Sever P, Thom S, eds. Cardiovascular Disease: Risk Factors and Intervention. Oxford: Radcliffe Press, 1993:47–52.

78. Stout RW. Insulin and atherogenesis. Eur J Epidemiol 1992; 8 (suppl 1):134–135.

79. Renard E, Bringer J, Jaffiol C. Steroides sexuels: Effets sur le metabolisme hydrocarboné avant et après la menopause. Presse Med 1993; 22:431–435.

80. Lindheim SR, Presser SC, Ditkoff EC, Vijod MA, Stanczyk FZ, Lobo RA. A possible bimodal effect of estrogen on insulin sensitivity in postmenopausal women and the attenuating effect of added progestin. Fertil Steril 1993; 60:664–647.

81. Nabulsi AA, Folsom AR, White A, Patsch W, Heiss G, Wu KK, Szklo M. Association of hormone-replacement therapy with various cardiovascular risk factors in postmenopausal women: The Atherosclerosis Risk in Communities Study Investigators. N Engl J Med 1993; 328:1069–1075.

82. Barrett-Connor E, Laakso M. Ischaemic heart disease risk in postmenopausal women: Effects of estrogen use on glucose and insulin levels. Arteriosclerosis 1990; 10:531–534.

83. Doyle JT, Dawber TR, Kannel WB, Heslin AS, Kahn HA. Cigarette smoking and coronary heart disease: Combined experience of the Albany and Framingham studies. N Engl J Med 1962; 266: 796–801.

84. Doll R, Peto R. Mortality in relation to smoking: 20 years observation of British doctors. Br Med J 1976; 4:152.

85. Fowler G. Smoking as a risk factor for cardiovascular disease. In: Poulter N, Sever P, Thom S, eds. Cardiovascular Disease: Risk Factors and Intervention. Oxford: Radcliffe Press, 1993:153–160.

86. Beard CM, Kottke TE, Annegers JF, Ballard DJ. The Rochester Coronary Heart Disease Project: Effect of cigarette smoking, hypertension, diabetes and steroidal estrogen use on coronary heart disease among 40- to 59-year old women, 1960 through 1982. Mayo Clin Proc 1989; 64: 1471–80.

87. Stampfer MJ. Smoking, estrogen and prevention of heart disease in women. Mayo Clin Proc 1989; 64:1553–1557.

88. Midgette AS, Baron JA. Cigarette smoking and the risk of natural menopause. Epidemiology 1990; 1:474–480.

89. Schlemmer A, Jensen J, Riis BJ, Christiansen C. Smoking induces androgen levels in early post-menopausal women. Maturitas 1990; 12:99–104.

90. Baron JA, La Vecchia C, Levi F. The antiestrogenic effect of cigarette smoking in women. Am J Obstet Gynecol 1990; 162:502–514.

91. Reid DD, Hamilton PJS, McCartney P, Rose G, Jarrett RJ, Keen H. Smoking and other risk factors for coronary heart disease in British civil servants. Lancet 1976; ii:979–984.

92. Rångemark C, Benthin G, Granström EF, Persson MT, Winell S, Wennmalm Å. Tobacco use and urinary excretion of thromboxane A2 and prostacyclin metabolites in women stratified by age. Circulation 1992; 86:1495–1500.

93. Grady D, Rubin SM, Petitti DB, Fox CS, Black D, Ettinger B, et al. Hormone therapy to prevent disease and prolong life in postmenopausal women. Ann Intern Med 1992; 117:1016–1037.

94. Stampfer MJ, Colditz GA, Willett WC, et al. Postmenopausal estrogen therapy and cardiovascular risk: ten year followup from the Nurses Health Study. N Engl J Med 1991; 325:756–762.

95. Wolf PH, Madans JH, Finucane FF, Higgins M, Kleinman JC. Reduction of cardiovascular disease-related mortality among postmenopausal women who use hormones: evidence from a national cohort. Am J Obstet Gynecol 1991; 164:489–494.

96. Lip GYH, Beevers DG, Zarifis J. Hormone Replacement Therapy and cardiovascular risk: the cardiovascular physicians' viewpoint. J Intern Med 1995. In press.

97. American College of Physicians. Guidelines for counselling postmenopausal women about preventive hormone therapy. Ann Intern Med 1992; 117:1038–1041.

98. Lip GYH, Beevers M, Churchill D, Beevers DG. Do clinicians prescribe hormone replacement therapy to hypertensive postmenopausal women? Br J Clin Prac 1995; 49:61–64.

99. Air A, Lip GYH, Beevers DG. Hormone replacement therapy: Attitudes of women should be considered (letter). Br Med J 1994; 309:192.

100. Piolte L, Hlatky M. Hormone replacement after menopause: importance of heart disease in women's decision making (abstr). J Am Coll Cardiol 1994; 23(suppl):51A.

101. Posthuma WFM, Westendorp RGJ, Vandenbroucke JP. Cardioprotective effect of hormone replacement therapy in postmenopausal women: is the evidence biased? Br Med J 1994; 308:1268–1269.

102. Khaw K-T, Peart WS. Blood pressure and contraceptive use. Br Med J 1982; 285:403–407.

103. Weir RJ, Briggs E, Mack A, Naismith L, Taylor L, Wilson E. Blood pressure in women taking oral contraceptives. Br Med J 1974; 1:533–535.

104. Christiansen C, Christensen MS, Hagen C, Stocklund KE, Transbøl I. Effects of natural estrogen/gestagen and thiazide on coronary risk factors in normal postmenopausal women. Acta Obstet Gynecol Scand 1981; 60:407–412.

105. Lind T, Cameron EC, Hunter WM, Leon C, Moran PF, Oxley A, Gerrard J, Lind UCG. A prospective controlled trial of six forms of hormone replacement therapy given to postmenopausal women. Br J Obstet Gynaecol 1979; 86(suppl 3):1–29.

106. Perry I, Beevers M, Beevers DG, Leusley D. Oestrogens and cardiovascular disease. Br Med J 1988; 297:1127.

107. Pfeffer RI, Kurosaki TT, Charlton SK. Estrogen use and blood pressure in later life. Am J Epidemiol 1979; 110:469–478.

108. von Eiff AW, Plotz EJ, Beck KJ, Czernik A. The effects of estrogens and progestins on blood pressure regulation of normotensive women. Am J Obstet Gynaecol. 1971; 4:31–47.

109. Barrett-Connor E, Wingard D, Criqui MH. Postmenopausal estro-

gen use and heart disease risk factors in the 1980s. JAMA 1989; 261:2095–2100.

110. Hammond CB, Jelovsek FR, Lee KL, Creasman WT, Parker RT. Effects of long-term estrogen replacement therapy. I. Metabolic effects. Am J Obstet Gynecol. 1979; 133:525–536.

111. Jespersen CM, Arnung K, Hagen C, Kilden T, Nielsen F, Nielsen MD, Giese J. Effects of natural oestrogen therapy on blood pressure and renin-angiotensin system in normotensive and hypertensive menopausal women. J Hypertens 1983; 1:361–364.

112. Lip GYH, Beevers M, Churchill D, Beevers DG. Hormone replacement therapy and blood pressure in hypertensive women. J Hum Hypertens 1994; 8:491–494.

113. Zarifis J, Lip GYH, Beevers DG. Discontinuing hormone replacement therapy and blood pressure in menopausal women with uncontrolled hypertension. Clin Sci 1995; 32(suppl):3P.

114. Meade TW, Chakrabarti R, Haines AP, Howarth DJ, North WRS, Stirling Y. Haemostatic, lipid and blood pressure profiles of women on oral contraceptives containing 50µg or 30mg oestrogen. Lancet 1977; ii:948–951.

115. Wallace RB, Hoover J, Barrett-Connor E, Rifkind BM, Hunninghake DB, Mackenthun A, Heiss G. Altered plasma lipid and lipoprotein levels associated with oral contraceptive and oestrogen use: report from the Medications Working Group of the Lipid Research Clinics Program. Lancet 1979; ii:112–115.

116. Varizi SM, Evans JC, Larson MG, Wilson PWF. The impact of female hormone usage on the lipid profile: The Framingham Offspring Study. Arch Intern Med 1993; 153:22006.

117. Wahl P, Walden C, Knopp R, Hoover J, Wallace R, Heiss G, Rifkind B. Effect of estrogen/progestin potency on lipid/lipoprotein cholesterol. N Engl J Med 1983; 308:862–867.

118. Barrett-Connor E, Bush TL. Estrogen and coronary heart disease in women. JAMA 1991; 265:1861–1867.

119. Bush TL, Barrett-Connor E, Cowan LD, Criqui MH, Wallace RB, Suchindran CM, et al. Cardiovascular mortality and non-contraceptive use of estrogen in women: results from the Lipid Research Clinics Program Follow-up Study. Circulation 1987; 75:1102–1109.

120. Stampfer MJ, Willett EC, Colditz GA, Rosner B, Speizer FE, Hennekens CH. A prospective study of postmenopausal estrogen therapy and coronary heart disease. N Engl J Med 1985; 313: 1044–1049.

121. Campos H, Wilson PW, Jimenez D, McNamara JR, Ordovas J, Schaefer EJ. Differences in apolipoproteins and low-density lipoprotein subfractions in postmenopausal women on and off estrogen therapy: results from the Framingham Offspring study. Metabolism 1990; 39:1033–1038.

122. Hirvonen E, Mälkönen M, Manninen V. Effects of different progestogens on lipoproteins during postmenopausal replacement therapy. N Engl J Med 1981; 304:560–563.

123. Montgomery JC, Crook D. Progestogens: symptomatic and metabolic side effects. In: Drife JO, Studd JWW, eds. HRT and Osteoporosis. London: Springer-Verlag, 1990:197–208.

124. Tikkanen MJ, Kuusi T, Nikkila EA, Sipinen S. Post-menopausal hormone replacement therapy: effects of progestogens on serum lipids and lipoproteins. Maturitas 1986; 8:7–17.

125. Soma MR, Osnag-Gadda I, Paoletti R, et al. The lowering of lipoprotein (a) induced by estrogen plus progesterone replacement therapy in postmenopausal women. Arch Intern Med 1993; 153:1462–1468.

126. Gambrell RD, Teran AZ. Changes in lipids and lipoproteins with long-term estrogen deficiency and hormone replacement therapy. Am J Obstet Gynecol 1991; 165:307–317.

127. Meilahn EN, Kuller LH, Matthews KA, Kiss JE. Hemostatic factors according to menopausal status and the use of hormone replacement therapy. Ann Epidemiol 1992; 2:445–455.

128. Garcia Rodriguez LA, Pfaff GM, Schumacher MC, Walker AM, Hoffmeister H. Replacement estrogen use and body mass index. Epidemiology 1990; 1:219–223.

7

Cardiovascular Complications and the Menopause

J. D. Swales

University of Leicester
and Leicester Royal Infirmary
Leicester, England

I. INTRODUCTION

Cardiovascular disease is the most important cause of mortality in the middle-aged and the elderly, exceeding even cancer in importance. The risk factors are fundamentally the same in all groups, although their relative importance differs. The major source of mortality is ischemic heart disease as a result of atheromatosis. The majority of strokes are also atheromatous—although a minority are due to hemorrhage, usually as a result of elevated blood pressure. Renal failure as a result of cardiovascular disease is usually a consequence of either hypertensive nephrosclerosis or renal arterial atheroma. Cardiac failure is usually a significant cause of death only in an age group older than that of the menopausal women, while peripheral vascular disease is also very uncommon in the absence of other predisposing risk factors.

II. ISCHEMIC HEART DISEASE

The incidence of cardiovascular disease in women is less than that in men for all age groups. In England and Wales, the annual incidence for coronary heart disease in men below the age of 65 was 88.6 per 100,000, while in women it was only 24.2 Even in older age groups (65–74 years) these differences are only moderately attenuated, with values of 1270 and 550, respectively (1). The gender difference is still preserved in hypertensives: In the Framingham study, the risk of cardiovascular disease in male hypertensives was approximately three times as great as in female hypertensives in all age strata (2). The risk ratio for hypertensives (compared with normotensives) was the same in both sexes, indicating that the difference in the incidence of cardiovascular disease could not be explained by blood-pressure differences.

Deaths from circulatory disease have declined in both men and women in the United Kingdom, Europe, Australasia, and the United States (3). The decline, however, has been much greater in women than men, and although it became apparent in men in the 1970s the decline has been observed in women over a much longer period. In the United States, for example, coronary heart disease mortality declined in females between 1886 and 1910 whereas in men coronary heart disease mortality increased until 1965 and then declined (4). While improved management of cardiovascular risk factors may have contributed to these changes, the reason for gender-specific effects remains unknown.

III. THE MENOPAUSE AND ISCHEMIC HEART DISEASE

The Framingham study provided evidence of other, more subtle gender differences in men and women (2). While the incidence rate of angina pectoris was similar in the two sexes, the incidence of more serious clinical manifestations, such as myocardial infarction and sudden death, was much lower in women. Athero-thrombotic brian infarction showed no clear male predominance.

Since the onset of menopause occurs at different ages, it is difficult to relate such epidemiological observations to the pre- or postmenopausal state. Accordingly, in further analysis, events were related to menopausal status. These data showed a twofold increase in cardiovascular-disease incidence among postmeno-pausal women compared with premenopausal women (2). The number of incidents was small, which limited the ability of the study to detect more specific effects. However, the relative risk of coronary heart disease in postmenopausal women seemed to be higher in the younger age strata (40–44 years) than in older groups. The fact that the difference in hormonal status between pre- and postmenopausal women is greatest in the younger age strata would support the view that differences in ischemic heart disease have a hormonal basis.

The pathology of ischemic heart disease is similar in both sexes. The differences in morbidity and mortality between men and women could therefore be due to a different risk factor profile or to differential cardiovascular response to risk factors. Hormonal changes associated with the menopause could con-tribute to both influences.

There is evidence that the impact of certain risk factors on the incidence of ischemic heart disease does differ. For instance, in a later analysis of the Framingham data (5), cigarette smoking was less important and blood glucose more important as predic-tors of subsequent ischemic heart disease in women.

Other small studies have provided support for the concept that the menopause increases the risk of coronary heart disease independent of age (6–11), but this observation has not been universally confirmed. In a large prospective cohort study of 121,700 U.S. women aged 30 to 55 years, Colditz et al. (12) specifi-cally addressed this point. The age-adjusted risk ratio was 1.7 (confidence limits 1.1 to 2.8). However, this fell to 1.0 when anal-yses controlled for age in 1-year rather than 5-year intervals and adjustment for cigarette smoking was made. The age- and smoking-adjusted risk ratio for patients undergoing a natural menopause was 1.2 (confidence limits 0.8 to 1.8). However, women who had undergone a surgical menopause with bilateral oophorectomy showed a significantly increased risk ratio of 2.2. The risk ratio fell to 0.8 in women who had subsequently been given estrogen replacement therapy. These data therefore supported the view that removal of endogenous estrogens by bilateral oophorectomy is a risk factor for cardiovascular disease that is reversible by estrogen therapy. An overview of published studies suggested that hormone replacement therapy for postmenopausal symptoms was associated with a reduction in risk of ischemic heart disease of about 25% in case-controlled studies and about 20% in prospective studies (13). One of the difficulties in discriminating cause and effect in the relationship between the menopause and ischemic heart disease is the interaction of factors. Clearly, age is the most important factor, but additionally smokers have an early menopause. However, conventional risk factors for cardiovascular disease are also of importance in menopausal women. Thus, in a study of the female residents of Rochester, Minnesota, aged between 40 and 59, cigarette smoking and hypertension were each associated with a fivefold increase of coronary heart disease, while diabetes was associated with an eightfold increase (14).

In addition, approximately two-thirds of all cases of myocardial infarction and sudden unexpected death in this group were associated with smoking, 45% with hypertension, and 13% with diabetes. In the best-documented study of risk-factor changes associated with the menopause, Matthews et al. (15) carried out a prospective investigation of 69 women who spontaneously stopped menstruating (aged 42–50 years) and 32 women who stopped menstruating and received hormone replacement therapy. In the absence of hormone replacement therapy, total and LDL cholesterol, triglycerides, apolipoproteins A1 and B, and fasting insulin and glucose increased and HDL cholesterol declined. Blood pressure did not change. In women who received hormone replacement therapy, although LDL did not increase, there was a substantial increase in triglycerides and apolipopro-tein AI.

In summary, the immediate effects of the menopause on the incidence of ischemic heart disease are small and difficult to dissociate from the normal increase in risk that occurs with age and the risks of smoking that are also associated with earlier menopause. Menopausal status per se does not seem to contrib-ute to the incidence of coronary artery disease, at least in the short term. The adverse effects of the menopause on risk factors for ischemic heart disease, however, may contribute to the longer-term increase in risk observed in menopausal women, although they never "catch up" with men in this respect, and the evidence from Framingham suggests a rather more benign pic-ture of ischemic heart disease that may reflect its development at a later age.

IV. STROKE AND RENAL FAILURE

Cohort studies on the association between ischemic heart disease and the menopause are too small to show an impact on stroke because the incidence of cerebrovascular disease is very low in relatively young women in the absence of other risk factors. This is even more true of renal failure, which exhibits an extremely low incidence in cohort studies. It seems likely, however, that the impact of the menopause on stroke incidence is even less than the impact on ischemic heart disease although, again, it is necessary to distinguish between effects related to aging and to the meno-pause per se.

The major risk factor for stroke is hypertension. Short-term cohort studies have demonstrated no effect of the menopause on blood pressure (15). Community-based epidemiological studies show a steady increase in systolic blood pressure with age in women that is steeper than the rise in men (16). Thus, the rate of rise in systolic blood pressure is 0.6–0.8 mm Hg per year for women compared with 0.3–0.5 mm Hg per year for men. By the seventh decade, blood pressure in women has "caught up" with that of men, but the point of crossover varies slightly among different studies in Western countries. After the 60s (for which data become much scarcer), women's systolic blood pressure usually exceeds that of men. A similar, but less steep, age-related rise in diastolic blood pressure is observed. There is no detectable change in gradient of either systolic or diastolic blood pressure in women at the common age for the menopause. The small and decreasing difference in both systolic and diastolic blood pressure between men and postmenopausal women would make a minimal and declining contribution to the risk of stroke. The weak association between plasma lipids and stroke (5) would indicate that menopausal changes in lipids would also be of less importance in the incidence of stroke than in that of ischemic heart disease. Epidemiological data support this view: In England and Wales, the incidence of stroke in men below the age of 65 was 14 per 100,000 compared with an incidence of 10.5 in women. Between the ages of 65 and 74, the figures were 295 and 220 per 100,000, respectively. The gender differences associated with ischemic heart disease were not observed with atherothrombotic infarction in the Framingham study (12). There is also evidence for attenuation of the gender-specific risks in high-risk patients, i.e., those with hypertension. In the MRC study of mild hypertension, while the risk of coronary events was 5- to 10-fold greater in men than in women at different ages, there were only small and variable differences in the risk of stroke, although the numbers were fairly small (17) (Table 1).

Hypertension is a risk factor for renal failure, and hypertensive renal disease is an important cause of end-stage dialysis-dependent renal failure. The decline in renal function in both middle-aged and elderly subjects is related to baseline blood pressure (18,19). In the only study to look specifically at gender differences, the impact of blood pressure on elevation of serum creatinine was slightly greater in men than in women (18). The small gender differences in menopausal women are unlikely to contribute significantly to the decline in renal function, and there is no clinical evidence that the menopause is important in this respect.

Table 1 Rates per 1000 Patients
Years of Observation in the MRC
Trial of Treatment in Mild
Hypertension

Age (yr)	Men	Women
Coronary rates		
35–44	3.3 (17)	0.3 (10)
45–54	8.7 (83)	1.1 (9)
55–64	13.4 (100)	2.6 (24)
Total	9.0 (200)	1.7 (34)
Stroke rates		
35–44	0.4 (2)	1.6 (5)
45–54	2.4 (23)	1.3 (11)
55–64	5.3 (40)	3.1 (28)
Total	2.9 (65)	2.1 (44)

Absolute numbers in parentheses.
Source: Adapted from Ref. 17.

V.   INTERMITTENT CLAUDICATION

Intermittent claudication is much less common in postmenopausal women than in men and is important as a cause of morbidity rather than mortality. However, it is an important predictor of cardiovascular mortality in its own right since it is
associated with atheroma elsewhere in the vascular tree. The
risk-factor profile is similar in both sexes—although in the
Framingham study, while cigarette smoking predominated,
obesity actually appeared to confer a slightly protective effect in
women (5).

REFERENCES

1.   Department of Health. Public Health Common Data Set 1993.
     Surrey, England: Institute of Public Health, 1993.

2. Kannel WB, Hjortland MC, McNamara PM, Gordon T. Menopause and risk of cardiovascular disease: The Framingham Study. Ann Intern Med 1976; 85:447–452.
3. Swales JD, Fletcher AE, Bulpitt CJ. Epidemiology. In: Messerli FH, ed. Cardiovascular Disease in the Elderly. 3rd ed. Boston: Kluwer, Academic Publishers, 1993.
4. Patrick CH, Palesch YY, Feinleib M, et al. Sex differences in declining cohort death rates from heart disease. Am J Pub Health, 1982; 72:161–166.
5. Stokes J, Kannel WB, Wolf PA, Cupples LA, D'Agostino B. The relative importance of selected risk factors for various manifestations of cardiovascular disease among men and women from 35 to 64 years old: 30 years of follow-up in the Framingham Study. Circulation 1987; 75(suppl V):V-65–V-73.
6. Rosenberg L, Hennekens CH, Rosner B, Belanger C, Rothman KJ, Speizer FE. Early menopause and the risk of myocardial infarction. Am J Obstet Gynecol 1981; 139:47–51.
7. Novec ER, Williams TJ. Autopsy comparison of cardiovascular changes in castrated and normal women. Am J Obstet Gynecol 1960; 80:863–872.
8. Wuest JH Jr, Dry TJ, Edwards JE. The degree of coronary atherosclerosis in bilaterally oophorectomised women. Circulation 1953; 7:801–809.
9. Bengtsson C. Ischaemic heart disease in women: a study based on a randomised population sample of women with myocardial infarction in Goteborg, Sweden. Acta Med Scand 1973; 549(suppl): 1–128.
10. Lindquist O. Influence of the menopause on ischaemic heart disease and its risk factors and on bone mineral content. Acta Obstet Gynecol Scand 1982; 110(suppl):17–21.
11. Parrish HM, Carr CA, Hall DG, King TM. Time interval from castration in premenopausal women to development of excessive coronary atherosclerosis. Am J Obstet Gynecol 1967; 99:155–162.
12. Colditz GA, Willett WC, Stampfer MJ, Rosner B, Speizer FE, Hennekens CH. Menopause and the risk of coronary heart disease in women. N Engl J Med 1987; 316:1105–1110.
13. Mead ETW, Berra A. Hormone replacement therapy and cardiovascular disease. Br Med Bull 1992; 48:276–304.
14. Beard M, Kottke TE, Annegers JF, Ballard DJ. The Rochester Coronary Heart Disease Project: Effect of cigarette smoking, hyperten-

sion, diabetes and steroidal estrogen use on coronary heart disease among 40- to 59-year-old women, 1960 through 1982. Mayo Clin Proc 1989; 64:1471–1480.

15. Matthews KA, Meilahn E, Kuller LH, Kelsey SF, Caggiula AW, Wing RR. Menopause and risk factors for coronary heart disease. N Engl J Med 1989; 321:641–646.

16. Whelton PK, He J, Klag MJ. Blood pressure in Westernised populations. In: Swales JD. Textbook of Hypertension. Oxford, England: Blackwell Scientific Publications, 1994:11–22.

17. Miall WE, Greenberg G. Mild Hypertension: Is There a Pressure to Treat? Cambridge, England: Cambridge University Press, 1987:111.

18. Perneger TV, Nieto J, Whelton PK, Klag MJ, Comstock GW, Szklo M. A prospective study of blood pressure and serum cretinine: Results from the "Clue" study and the ARIC study. JAMA 1993; 269:488–493.

19. Lindeman RD, Tobin JD, Shock NW. Association between blood pressure and the rate of decline in renal function with age. Kidney Int 1984; 26:861–868.

8

Lipids, Hormone Replacement Therapy, and Diet

Coronary Heart Disease in Postmenopausal Women

Veronica Ravnikar and Brenda Kramer-Coutinho

University of Massachusetts Medical Center
Worcester, Massachusetts

I. INTRODUCTION

Cardiovascular disease is the most common cause of death in the United States and other developed countries. It includes coronary heart disease (CHD), hypertension, peripheral vascular disease, and strokes. Diseases of the heart are the leading cause of death in women in the United States, resulting in approximately 250,000 deaths each year and 500,000 deaths each year for all cardiovascular diseases together (1). Numerous studies have shown that, in general, cardiovascular disease in women occurs about 10–12 years later in life than in men. For example, the incidence of CHD in men 35 to 44 years old is over three times higher than in age-matched women; by the age of 65 to 74 years, the incidence is the same for men and women (2).

The incidence of CHD in women has a striking relationship to menopause. After controlling for other risk factors, post-menopausal women have higher rates of CHD and myocardial infarction (MI) than do premenopausal women of the same age (3). Incidence of MI is negligible in premenopausal women and is related to cigarette smoking, use of high-dose estrogen oral contraceptive agents, hypertension, diabetes, or dyslipidemia (4).

During the reproductive years, women are "protected" from CHD. A review of the literature shows overwhelming evidence for a reduced risk of cardiovascular disease in post-menopausal women receiving estrogen replacement therapy, and there are many excellent review articles illustrating the relationship between hormone replacement therapy and atherosclerotic risk (5–8). More specifically, data from prospective longitudinal studies such as the Leisure World Study, the Lipid Research Clinics Follow-up, the National Health and Nutrition Examination Survey Epidemiologic Follow-up Study (NHANES I), and, more recently, the Nurses' Health Study support a 40–60% reduction in cardiovascular-disease risk in postmenopausal patients currently using estrogen replacement therapy (9–13). Only one of the large studies addressing this issue found an increased risk of cardiovascular disease in estrogen users. The Framingham Heart Study, presenting data in 1978 and 1985, argued that there was a 50% increased risk for cardiovascular disease in estrogen users. The impact of this finding could not be ignored because of the enormous respect accorded the Framingham study; however, in a subsequent reanalysis of the data, the authors reversed their conclusion when they eliminated angina as an endpoint (14,15). Table 1 summarizes these large cohort studies of estrogen use and cardiovascular disease.

It is now generally accepted that physiological levels of estrogen are "cardioprotective" and that postmenopausal estrogen replacement therapy (ERT) decreases the risk of cardiovascu-

Table 1 Summary of Large[a] Cohort Studies of Estrogen Use in Women and Cardiovascular Disease (CVD)

Author	n	Endpoint	Risk estimate
Bush (1987)	2,270	CVD death	0.34[b]
Stampfer (1991)	48,470	CHD	0.51[b]
Henderson (1988)	8,807	MI	0.54[b]
Petitti (1987)	3,437	All CVD	0.60
Wolf (1991)	1,944	Fatal CVD	0.66[b]
Avila (1990)	24,900	Nonfatal MI	0.70
Wilson (1985)	1,234	All CVD	1.76[b]

CHD = coronary heart disease.
MI = myocardial infarction.
[a]Sample size >1000 women.
[b]Statistically significant.
Source: Ref. 21.

lar mortality by approximately 50%. The reasons for this "protection" during the reproductive years are complex, but a significant factor is the higher high-density lipoprotein (HDL) levels and lower low-density lipoprotein (LDL) levels in premenopausal women. The focus of the assessment of cardiovascular risk and intervention with hormone replacement therapy for postmenopausal women has traditionally been on plasma lipoprotein levels. While LDL and total cholesterol levels do increase after menopause (16), and estrogen has been shown to reverse these changes in addition to increasing HDL cholesterol, this is probably a narrow view of the cardioprotection mechanism of estrogen. It has been pointed out that the degree of protection is greater than can be attributed statistically to the lipoprotein profile and that only 25–50% of the cardioprotective effect of estrogen can be explained by lipoprotein concentrations (8,12). Thus, the protection not mediated by lipoproteins is growing in importance.

In addition to elevated blood lipid levels, obesity and hypertension are also major risk factors for cardiovascular disease in women. Fortunately, these risk factors may be responsive to lifestyle-change intervention.

It is the purpose of this chapter to: 1) provide the background necessary to understand the physiology of lipoproteins and how they are affected by estrogens and progestins, 2) review the impact of hormone replacement therapy on serum lipoproteins, and 3) discuss nutrition and exercise intervention in the postmenopausal woman.

II. A BRIEF REVIEW OF LIPOPROTEIN PHYSIOLOGY

Plasma cholesterol is a risk factor for heart disease in both sexes. Over 90% of total cholesterol in the serum is carried by two major lipoproteins: LDL and HDL cholesterols. Lipoprotein physiology is based on concepts of lipoprotein particles and their interactions with one another, with cells, and with interstitial components. Lipoproteins are classified by the density of salt solution at which they begin to float, hence, very low-density lipoprotein (VLDL), LDL, and HDL. These particles can also be conceptualized by size, with VLDL and chylomicrons having relatively large diameters (70–200 nm), LDL being an intermediate size (20–27 nm), and HDL being relatively small (8–13 nm) (18).

Two large particle systems are used for triglyceride distribution in the body: one that originates in the liver (VLDL) and is eventually converted into the long-lived particle (LDL) and another that originates in the small intestine and is completely removed by either the liver or bone marrow (chylomicrons). The surface proteins of these particles ultimately determine their functions, as either enzymes or cofactors, or via specific interaction with cell-surface receptors or with the other particles. Each of the two large particle systems has a characteristic apoprotein on its surface that remains attached to the particle. These apoproteins, apo B-100 and apo B-48, have a central role in lipoprotein physiology, and apo B-100 plays an especially important role in the development of atherosclerosis. Apo B-48 particles (chylomicrons) are stuffed with triglycerides but, unlike the apo B-100 particles, they are rapidly taken up after each meal by the liver and bone marrow and are short-lived. Apo B-100 particles start out on the surface of VLDLs, which are stuffed with triglycerides and cholesterol, and function to deliver triglycerides to tissues of the body. Triglycerides are removed from these particles by the action of lipoprotein lipase, an enzyme on the surface of endothelial cells. As the triglycerides are distributed from these particles, they grow progressively smaller, more dense, and more cholesterol-rich, and—still retaining the B-100 apoprotein—they are then called LDL particles.

LDLs are long-lived and serve as the body's source of cholesterol. Cells of the body take up these particles by placing LDL receptors on their surface. It is these apo B-100, LDL particles that are referred to as "bad" cholesterol, because they can be modified in such a way that macrophages within vessel walls consume them and transform into foam cells, the microscopic hallmark of atherosclerosis. One of the mechanisms of LDL modification resulting in atherosclerosis seems to be oxidation (18).

Another particle has recently received attention as being critically important in the development of atherosclerosis: an apo B-100 particle that has an additional protein linked to its surface. It is referred to as lipoprotein (a) or Lp(a), and it has a strong association with atherosclerosis. Unlike other lipoproteins, Lp(a) appears to be resistant to most conventional treatments for hyperlipidemia and is an independent risk factor for atherosclerosis when serum concentrations are above 30 mg/dl (19). Furthermore, this particle is not measured by the assays currently used to measure total cholesterol, triglycerides, and HDLs. It has even been suggested that there may be an age-related increase in this lipoprotein in postmenopausal women (reviewed in Ref. 19).

The small particle system refers to HDL, or "good" cholesterol. Briefly, HDL cholesterol seems to function against the development of atherosclerosis by serving as an exchangeable apoprotein buffer, in reverse cholesterol transport carrying cholesterol from cells such as macrophage foam cells back to the liver, and as a buffer for removing excess lipids during lipolysis.

III. EFFECTS OF ESTROGEN ON LIPOPROTEINS

The effect of estrogen on plasma lipoproteins appears to be mediated in at least four distinct ways. First, estrogen appears to increase the hepatic production of VLDLs. It also increases the removal of the long-lived, cholesterol-rich LDL particle. It appears to do this by increasing the activity of the LDL receptors in the liver. Taken together, these mechanisms point to the observation that estrogen increases the flux of apo B-100 through the plasma by increasing both production and removal (20). The third mechanism is through inhibition of an enzyme found on the endothelial surface of the liver, hepatic lipase (HL). This enzyme is similar to lipoprotein lipase, the enzyme responsible for removing triglycerides from VLDLs and chylomicrons in the circulation, except that HL appears to act on LDLs and HDLs and not VLDLs and chylomicrons. Hepatic lipase action on HDLs may be primarily on the larger, less dense HDL called HDL-2. HDL-2 is thought to be better correlated with protection from heart disease (18). If HL acts on HDL-2 and the triglycerides are removed, the resultant HDLs will become smaller and denser: HDL-3. The result of estrogen's inhibition of HL is to leave some triglycerides in the apo B-100 particles, which may leave more particles available for the liver's LDL receptor to finally remove from the circulation. Also, HL inhibition by estrogen would lead to more HDL-2. Lastly, estrogen seems to decrease Lp(a), although whether the mechanism is decreased synthesis or increased removal is unclear at this time (18).

IV. NONLIPID EFFECTS OF ESTROGEN

As mentioned, it appears that only 25–50% of the cardioprotective action of estrogen may be directly related to lipoproteins. Although many clinicians still believe that estrogen raises blood pressure—probably reflecting older data with high-dose estrogen oral contraceptives—most clinical trials of noncontraceptive estrogen have found that postmenopausal women assigned to ERT tend to have lower blood pressure than untreated women (21). Estrogen appears to exert a protective effect directly on the arterial wall independent of circulating lipoproteins. The presence of estrogen and progestin receptors in arterial endothelium and smooth muscle lends support to this theory of direct action. Several studies performed in monkeys suggest that estrogen modifies the constrictor responses of atherosclerotic coronary arteries and that, in a postmenopausal model in these monkeys, estrogen alone or estrogen with progesterone in a sequential manner significantly reduced atherosclerosis independently of the lipoprotein profile. A direct inhibition of LDL accumulation and an increase in LDL metabolism in arterial vessels could be demonstrated in these monkeys being fed an atherogenic diet (reviewed in Ref. 5).

In another study (22), administration of estrogen to cholesterol-fed rabbits dramatically retarded arterial lesion development despite its lack of effect on plasma cholesterol concentration and lipoprotein profile. In addition to the effects on lipoproteins and a direct antiatherosclerotic effect in arteries, other possible beneficial actions of estrogens on cardiovascular disease include: augmentation of vasodilating and antiplatelet aggregation factors, both endothelium-dependent (nitric oxide and prostacyclin) and endothelium-independent mechanisms, direct inotropic actions on the heart, improvement of peripheral glucose metabolism with a subsequent decrease in circulating insulin levels, and inhibition of lipoprotein oxidation (5).

V. EFFECTS OF PROGESTIN ON LIPOPROTEINS AND THE USE OF COMBINED ESTROGEN–PROGESTIN REPLACEMENT THERAPY

The addition of a progestin to estrogen replacement therapy is now recommended in postmenopausal women with an intact uterus to protect the endometrium from estrogen-induced hyperplasia and cancer. The risk of endometrial cancer in women receiving unopposed estrogens is approximately 2–10 times greater than that in untreated women (5). Unfortunately, it is well known that progestins, in general, attenuate the effects of estrogens on lipoproteins. Most of the data in the literature raise concern that progestins negate the positive effect of estrogen on HDLs. Androgenic progestins, including the 19-C nortestosterone derivatives such as norgestrel, increase HL activity and therefore decrease HDL cholesterol. The less androgenic agents— for example, the (21-C) 17-alpha-hydroxyprogesterone derivatives such as medroxyprogesterone acetate (MPA)—used most often in HRT in the United States appear to stimulate HL to a lesser degree, thus inducing a smaller decrease in HDLs (23).

Tables 2 and 3, taken from a review article by Barrett-Connor and Miller in 1993 (21), summarizes the lipid effects of conjugated equine estrogen at a 0.625 mg/day dose versus the lipid effects of conjugated equine estrogen at 0.625 mg/day and medroxyprogesterone acetate at different dosages either cyclically or continuously administered. Progestins do not appear to change the levels of LDL cholesterol significantly (24,25). Instead of the 13–16% increase in HDLs with unopposed estrogen, the studies of progestin combined with estrogen regimens (PERT) showed a variable decrease in HDLs, probably depend-

Table 2 Lipid Effects of Conjugated Equine Estrogen 0.625 mg Daily

Author	n	Duration (mo)	(% Change) HDL-C	LDL-C
Farish (1986)	21	6	16.0	−5.0
Sonnendecker (1989)	10	6	13.8	−19.7
Sherwin (1990)	27	12	13.7	0.3
Miller (1991)	31	4	14.0	−13.0
Walsh (1991)	31	3	16.0	−15.0

HDL = high-density lipoprotein.
LDL = low-density lipoprotein.
Source: Ref. 21.

Table 3 Lipid Effects of Conjugated Equine Estrogen 0.625 mg and Medroxyprogesterone Acetate (MPA)

Author	n	Duration (mo)	MPA dose (mg/day)	(% Change) HDL-C	(% Change) LDL-C
Cyclical administration					
Sherwin (1990)	25	12	5	4.3	−3.4
Miller (1991)	32	8	10	0.0	−14.0
Prough (1987)	10	9	10	24.6	−10.8
Weinstein (1990)	12	3	5	11.0	−17.6
Clisham (1991)	11	3	10	2.0	−18.0
Kable (1990)	22	3	5	7.2	−24.6
Continuous administration					
Weinstein (1990)	12	3	2.5	3.7	−21.0
	12	3	5.0	3.5	−18.6
Prough (1987)	16	9	2.5	12.7	−1.5
Clisham (1991)	11	3	10.0	2.0	−18.0
Kable (1990)	20	3	2.5	0.25	−11.5
Kable (1990)	18	3	5.0	4.7	−23.0

Source: Ref. 21.

ing on when in the cycle the serum was drawn, differences between laboratories, the amount of progestin prescribed, and for how long. Conclusions regarding the impact of progestational agents on cardiovascular disease are very much influenced by dose and duration of administration of the progestin. It seems that, while short-term studies suggest a negative impact of progestin, long-term studies indicate that this short-term effect disappears (5).

In other studies, no significant change in HDL levels was seen with ERT versus PERT, and levels were higher than those in untreated controls. For example, Barrett-Connor and coworkers (26), who studied postmenopausal women in Rancho Bernardo, California, found that the women using both estrogen and progestin (0.625 mg/day for at least 20 days with MPA 10 mg/day for 7–14 days each month) demonstrated the same favorable impact on cardiovascular risk factors (increased HDLs, decreased LDLs, and decreased blood pressure) that estrogen-only users did, when compared to the nonusers. Data from a cross-sectional study by Gambrell and Teran in 1991 (29) indicated that the progestogens—even the androgenic progestogens—did not negate the estrogen-induced increase in HDLs and decrease in LDLs over the long term, as their follow-up was from 1 to 44 years. More recently, in 1993, Nabulsi et al. (27) reported that users of estrogen with progestin and users of estrogen alone had similar levels of HDLs, HDL-2, HDL-3, cholesterol, apo A-I, LDLs, apo B, and Lp(a). However, this study is limited somewhat by its cross-sectional data and an inability to evaluate associations between variables and hormones according to the type, dose, duration of use, and mode of administration, especially in former users.

Soma and colleagues (19) reported not only a 30% decreased LDL level and a 19% increased HDL level in patients using a PERT regimen of 1.25 mg/day conjugated estrogen and MPA 10 mg/day for 10 days a month for 12 months, but also a 50% decrease in Lp(a) levels. As previously discussed, Lp(a) is a relatively recently described cardiovascular risk factor that is not usually measured in standard lipoprotein-cholesterol-measurement assays. The possibility that HRT may lower its level may have profound implications for the public health benefit of HRT, especially in patients with familial CHD and increased levels of this lipoprotein, which is usually resistant to most environmental influences and lifestyle factors (28).

A major obstacle to fully understanding the impact of ERT and PERT on lipid profiles and, more importantly, on cardiovascular endpoints is not only the lack of long-term, controlled, prospective studies but also the difficulty in analyzing the existing literature because of differences in dosages, preparations, routes of administration, and duration of therapy. Studies with the continuously administered combination of an estrogen and a low-dose progestational agent are emerging and reporting a favorable impact on lipid profile. One such study is from Weinstein et al. (30), who documented favorable changes in both HDLs and LDLs in women on 0.625 mg/day and either 2.5 mg or 5.0 mg of

MPA for 1 year. Christiansen and Riis (31) have documented the maintenance of a favorable lipid profile over 5 years of treatment with continuous combined estradiol and 1 mg norethindrone acetate. Studies currently underway, such as PEPI (the Postmenopausal Estrogen Progestins Trial) and the Women's Health Initiative, should provide more prospective data. (See Note Added in Proof, p. 169.)

VI. CARDIOVASCULAR RISK FACTORS AND HRT: A SUMMARY

The average American woman will live one-third of her life after the onset of the climacteric, and it has become accepted that hormone replacement therapy is appropriate for many women in this phase of their lives. HRT significantly decreases the risk of cardiovascular disease and osteoporosis, and provides relief from symptoms such as vasomotor hot flushes and urogenital atrophy that affect quality of life. Evidence is accumulating that there is a progestational dose that protects the endometrium but avoids a significant negating effect of the benefits of estrogen on lipoprotein profile. In addition, with a growing appreciation of the beneficial impact of estrogen independent of the lipoprotein profile, the addition of the progestin is a source of slightly less concern.

It is important to understand that small changes in lipoprotein profiles may have major effects on CHD. The Lipid Research Clinics Trial (12) demonstrated that a 1% reduction in cholesterol level equaled a 2% reduction in CHD, and an 11% decrease in LDL cholesterol levels resulted in a 19% decrease in CHD. A 1 mg/dl increase in HDL may be associated with a 3–5% decrease in CHD (32). Consequently, it is important to investigate methods other than HRT to improve the lipoprotein profile of the postmenopausal woman. Other risk factors for CHD that affect lipoprotein profiles are smoking and obesity, especially central adiposity. Gambrell and Teran (29) noted in their 1991 study that obesity and smoking affected lipids more than progestogens did in estrogen users. Greater weight yielded higher mean values of total cholesterol and LDL cholesterol and lower levels of HDL cholesterol. Smoking depressed HDLs and increased total cholesterol and LDLs in untreated women, even slightly more than in the hormone-user group.

In the remainder of this chapter we address the effects of nutritional intervention, weight loss, and physical activity on the lipoprotein profiles of postmenopausal women.

VII. THE ROLE OF NUTRITION IN LIPID PROFILE IMPROVEMENT AND CHD PREVENTION

As they age, many women and men require dietary intervention for elevated blood cholesterol levels; approximately 50% of all women aged 55 to 74 years are candidates for intervention (4). It has long been recognized that an elevated plasma cholesterol is a major risk factor for CHD. Diet significantly affects plasma cholesterol, and it is well established that diet is important in the prevention and treatment of elevated plasma lipid levels (33). Two excellent articles on common sources and effect on plasma lipids of major dietary fatty acids and the chemistry of their fatty-acid composition are a report of the National Cholesterol Education Program (33) and a review article by Grundy and Denke (35). Saturated fatty acids (e.g., coconut or palm oil, beef) and cholesterol in the diet raise levels of plasma cholesterol whereas polyunsaturated fatty acids (omega-6) lower them.

Among the proposed mechanisms by which saturated fatty acids and cholesterol affect plasma lipids are: decreasing hepatic LDL receptor synthesis and activity (including compositional changes in VLDLs and HDLs so that they become enriched in apo E and cholesterol esters and subsequently may bind to the LDL receptor), increasing all lipoprotein fractions, and decreasing chylomicron size (33). Mechanisms by which polyunsaturated fatty acids may favorably affect the lipid profile include: increasing fecal steroid and bile salt excretion, inducing compositional changes in LDLs and other lipoproteins that alter their metabolism, decreasing hepatic VLDL synthesis, increasing fractional catabolism of apo A-I and A-II, and decreasing synthesis and increasing catabolism of apolipoproteins (33).

In recent years, the media and the supplement industry have made much of the importance of the omega-3 fatty acids that are provided by fish and fish oils. These have been shown to lower plasma triglycerides and, to a lesser extent, plasma total cholesterol levels. Mechanisms by which fish oil affects plasma lipid levels include reduced synthesis of VLDLs and LDLs as well as increased HDL receptors and turnover of HDLs (which may actually lead to decreased plasma levels of HDL). Omega-3 fatty acids may also be antithrombotic through their effect on platelets and endothelial cells. Therefore, these fatty acids may also decrease CVD risk via mechanisms other than their effects on lipid profile (33).

Unfortunately, investigators have been able to show this relationship only with 90–120 g/day of fish oil, which is a level far in excess of amounts that could habitually be included in the diet (33). Consequently, recommendations about a realistic intake of fish oil and its effects on plasma cholesterol cannot be made at this time.

Monounsaturated fatty acids have also been shown to lower plasma total cholesterol and LDL levels when substituted for saturated fatty acids in the diet. A study by Mensink and Katan in 1989 (34) concluded that a mixed diet rich in monounsaturated fat (e.g., olive oil) was as effective as a diet rich in polyunsaturated fat (e.g., sunflower oil, corn oil) in lowering LDL cholesterol. Interestingly, both diets lowered the level of HDL cholesterol slightly in men but not in women.

In another study, Mata and coworkers (36) investigated the effects of diets rich in monounsaturated fat and polyunsaturated fat in pre- and postmenopausal women. Although the sample size was small, they concluded that diets rich in monounsaturated fats are as efficient as diets rich in polyunsaturated fats in decreasing LDL cholesterol regardless of menopausal status.

Studies demonstrate a lowering of plasma total cholesterol and LDL levels in patients on diets in which monounsaturated fatty acids were substituted for saturated fatty acids. However, HDL levels are unaffected or lowered (33).

Unresolved issues are: whether reduction of HDL levels by diet will increase the risk of atherosclerosis and whether the decrease negates any of the beneficial effect of decreasing LDL levels, or whether dietary reduction of serum HDLs is benign. The last is an interesting question because certain populations in the world that consume low-fat, high-complex-carbohydrate diets have low levels of both LDLs and HDLs and also have low rates of CHD (4,35). While the decrease in HDLs may not seem favorable—especially in women, in whom the level of HDL is such a strong risk factor—some workers conclude that diet-induced decreases in HDLs may not enhance coronary risk (35).

Other dietary factors that favorably affect plasma lipid levels are soluable fiber and vegetarianism. Coffee consumption has been shown to have both an association and a causal relationship with plasma lipid levels. However, findings from studies investigating this have been inconsistent. Some investigators suggest limiting coffee intake to one to two cups a day, while others report that CHD risk increases significantly when intake exceeds nine cups a day (33). Therefore, specific recommendations for coffee intake may be premature at this time, although moderation appears prudent. Epidemiological and clinical studies have shown a protective effect of moderate alcohol consumption on the incidence of CHD and a favorable effect of alcohol on HDL levels. However, recommendations to increase alcohol intake seem quite inappropriate in view of its abuse potential and link to other diseases, such as cirrhosis and breast cancer.

Interest in the antioxidant vitamin E as a nutrient protective against CHD has intensified recently with the recognition that oxidized LDLs may be involved in atherogenesis, as previously mentioned. Stampfer and colleagues (37) studied the association between vitamin E intake and the incidence of major coronary disease events in the Nurses' Health Study, which followed 87,245 female nurses 34 to 59 years of age for 8 years using dietary questionnaires. They found a statistically significant reduction in the risk of major coronary disease in women with a high intake of vitamin E (>200 IU/day) as compared with those with a low intake. This risk reduction was approximately 40%. The apparent benefit was attributable to the use of vitamin E supplements, since high levels of intake from dietary sources were not associated with significant reductions in risk. In addition, users of vitamin E for less than 2 years had no significant reductions in risk. It is suggested that public-policy recommendations concerning vitamin E intake await results of randomized trials of adequate size, such as the Women's Health Study.

In summary, dietary recommendations to decrease total cholesterol and LDL cholesterol include changing from a typical daily American diet to one with less than 30% of its calories from fat, with less than 10% of calories from saturated fatty acids, and less than 300 mg of cholesterol. This regimen should lower plasma total cholesterol by 5–7%, and even more in individuals with hypercholesterolemia. Reducing saturated fatty acids to less than 7% and cholesterol to less than 200 mg daily will lower total cholesterol by 10–20%. Further dietary modifications, such as increasing soluble fiber, may lead to additional reductions in plasma cholesterol of 1–10% (33). A recent study (38) has shown that dietary changes required to meet current dietary recommendations are relatively simple and do not require eliminating food groups and/or using special foods or products.

Table 4 shows the percentage of women meeting contemporary dietary recommendations in 1991 (4). Although women were included in a number of studies that examined diet-lipid relationships, many of these pooled data, and therefore gender effects, cannot be readily assessed. The questions that need to be addressed are whether dietary responsiveness in terms of effects on lipid profile are similar in men and in women, as well as whether there are differences in effects between pre- and postmenopausal women.

Table 4 Percentage of Women Meeting Contemporary Dietary
Recommendations

Recommendation	Age (yr)				
	30–39	40–49	50–59	60–69	>70
≤30% of energy from fat	15	15	18	20	19
≤10% of energy from saturated fatty acids	14	16	23	21	20
<300 mg cholesterol per day	72	75	70	74	81
>55% of energy from carbohydrate	16	18	13	17	23
≈25 g fiber per day	2	<1	5	1	2

Dietary recommendations derived from unpublished data from the International Life
Sciences Research Foundation, Washington, D.C., 1991.
Source: Ref. 4.

VIII. EFFECTS OF OBESITY, WEIGHT LOSS, AND PHYSICAL ACTIVITY ON THE LIPID PROFILE

Obesity was shown to be a significant independent predictor for
cardiovascular disease in the Framingham Study. In general,
obesity is associated with a more atherogenic lipoprotein profile,
and it has been shown that for each percentage of increase in
relative body-fat weight, a 1.1 mg/dl increase in serum cholesterol can be predicted (33). Results of the Gothenburg Population
Study (reviewed in Ref. 33) have shown that the anthropometric
indicator of waist-to-hip ratio (WHR) was associated most
strongly with the incidence of ischemic heart disease, especially
in women.

Dattilo and Kris-Etherton (39) performed a meta-analysis of
over 70 studies to quantify effects of weight loss by dieting on
lipids and lipoproteins. This was undertaken because the literature supporting the effects of weight loss on lipids and lipoproteins has been inconsistent. Results from the meta-analysis indicated that weight reduction was associated with significant
decreases in total cholesterol, LDLs, VLDLs, and triglycerides.

Each kilogram of weight loss was associated with a 0.05 mmol/L decrease in total cholesterol and a 0.02 mmol/L decrease in LDL. The overall probability for determining whether a relationship between weight reduction and HDL levels existed, however, was not significant for the total sample. When findings for HDLs were subgrouped into those at active and stabilized weight-loss periods, significant results emerged. A decrease in HDLs of 0.09 mmol/L was associated with active weight loss and a 0.14 mmol/L increase in HDLs was associated with a reduced, stabilized weight.

A mechanism responsible for this phenomenon has been proposed. Lipoprotein lipase activity generally increases with weight loss, especially once weight stabilizes. However, during acute energy restriction, tissue concentrations of lipoprotein lipase have been reported to decrease by 50–80% (39). Because of the decreased enzyme activity during active weight loss, triglyceride-rich lipoprotein synthesis is diminished and VLDL catabolism impaired; thus, transfer of lipids to HDLs is limited, leading to decreased HDL levels. When weight is stabilized at a reduced level, lipoprotein lipase has been reported to increase with the opposite effect, thereby increasing HDL levels. An important point is that, because subjects in these studies lost weight, it is possible that the intake of total dietary fat, saturated fatty acids, and cholesterol simultaneously decreased. Therefore, in this meta-analysis it is impossible to determine the independent influence of dietary fat on changes in lipids and lipoproteins.

In any case, it is clear that weight control is important in CHD risk management. Regression analysis also indicated that sex was significantly related to the change in HDLs and triglycerides. Men showed greater changes in triglycerides and HDL cholesterol. Age of subjects was also related to the change in LDLs with weight loss: Younger subjects (average, 34 years) showed an approximate fourfold difference in the decrease in LDLs with weight reduction compared to older subjects (average, 46 years). This is interesting because, as individuals age, LDLs usually increase; however, initial LDL level was not related to the change in LDLs with weight loss. Unfortunately, the meta-analysis reported no conclusions about the effects of weight loss on the lipid profile in pre- versus postmenopausal women.

Anderson and coworkers (40) published a study in 1990 that examined obese young and postmenopausal women before and during a prolonged period of treatment with low-energy intake under strictly standardized conditions. The study included 36 premenopausal and 68 postmenopausal women prescribed an 1100 kcal/day diet consisting of 27% protein, 18% fat, and 56% carbohydrate. The results showed that, while both groups exhibited a 5% decrease in baseline body weight, younger women appear to lose less fat than postmenopausal women; perhaps, the authors suggest, this is due to the relative difficulty in mobilization of the large gluteal femoral fat deposits. They concluded that younger women may encounter more difficulties in losing fat on diets, which may be due to the fact that they readily mobilize only a certain proportion of their adipose tissue, while other sites may be protected.

Exercise is generally accepted as a mechanism to increase HDL levels in men. Although cross-sectional studies confirm that active women have higher HDL levels than sedentary women, intervention studies in women have not consistently shown that HDL levels rise with exercise-training programs in the absence of other interventions (41). In the Lipid Research Clinics Follow-up Study, HDL level was the major lipid predictor of cardiovascular mortality in women (12). Does exercise increase HDL levels in women? In postmenopausal women? Despite the prevailing belief that exercise does increase HDL levels in women, very few studies have been performed in this population. Existing studies have methodological problems, such as lack of a control group or failure to consider confounding factors such as menopausal status, use of hormonal therapy, dietary composition, and change in weight.

Additional factors that should be considered when evaluating exercise-training studies are the duration and type of exercise, as well as exercise intensity and frequency. Of critical importance is documenting efficacy of exercise endpoints such as an increase in maximum oxygen consumption and resting metabolic rate. The effects on HDL levels of a 2-year walking program were evaluated in a randomized trial of 204 postmenopausal women who were not receiving hormone replacement therapy. The exercise volume in the study was low, approximately 11.2 km weekly, and training efficacy was not documented. After controlling for obesity, smoking, alcohol consumption, and compliance, the exercise intervention produced no change in HDL levels (41). A study was performed in which 17 postmenopausal women not receiving HRT were trained for 8 months in a regimen consisting of a walk–jog protocol for 45 minutes, three times per week, with no change in the composition of the subjects' diet. Despite an increase in maximum oxygen consumption and a decrease in body fat, there were no significant changes in plasma total cholesterol or HDL levels in either the exercise or the control group (41).

More recently, Svendsen and colleagues (42) studied the effect of exercise added to an energy-restrictive diet in overweight postmenopausal women. In a longitudinal clinical study, 121 healthy, overweight, postmenopausal women were randomly assigned to three groups: controls, those on a 4200 kJ/day diet, or those on a 4200 kJ/day diet with combined aerobic and anaerobic exercise. Body composition, fat distribution, resting metabolic rate, blood pressure, and serum lipoproteins and lipids were measured before and after 12 weeks of intervention. All the women in the intervention groups lost weight, and those on the diet-plus-exercise regimen increased their cardiopulmonary capacity. Serum triglycerides, total cholesterol, LDLs, VLDLs, and systolic blood pressure all significantly and equally decreased in both intervention groups compared to controls. Thus, in this study, there was a profound decrease in all risk factors for CVD that was similar whether or not exercise was added to the diet. However, the addition of combined aerobic and anaerobic exercises to an energy-restrictive diet promoted the loss of fat and preserved the lean-tissue mass in overweight postmenopausal women.

In a study of premenopausal, mildly obese women, Nieman and coworkers (43) compared diet with diet-plus-exercise for effects on serum lipids and lipoproteins. Both groups of women consumed 1258 kcal/day lactovegetarian diets while the diet-plus-exercise group walked at 60% heart-rate reserve during 45-minute sessions, five times per week for 5 weeks. Although exercise improved maximum oxygen consumption, changes in total body weight, lean body weight, and fat weight did not differ between groups. Both groups also had similar decreases in total cholesterol, LDLs, triglycerides, and glucose. There were, however, significant differences between groups in the pattern of change in serum HDL levels. It was concluded that the effect of moderate exercise on indices of serum lipid and lipoproteins is limited to HDL cholesterol.

In summary, then, there are not sufficient data to demonstrate that exercise training has an important independent effect on HDL levels in postmenopausal women. Exercise training in older women may attenuate the age-related increase in total cholesterol and the HDL-lowering effects of a fat-restricted low-energy diet (41). It is important to note, however, that postmenopausal women who exercise as well as diet may benefit from a decreased risk of falls, fractures, and all-cause mortality due to improved physical fitness and sense of well-being.

IX. RESEARCH QUESTIONS

There are many research questions to be answered with respect to the prevention of coronary heart disease in women. First, we need to understand the metabolic, cellular, and molecular bases for CHD, particularly how they may differ from the mechanisms in men. Other specific research questions that emerge include: What factors affect plasma lipids in women? How does risk-factor modification affect CHD in women of all ages, post-menopausal women, and those receiving hormone replacement therapy? Is it important to prevent or attenuate the decrease in HDL level in response to a low-fat diet? How is risk-factor modification affected by age, menopausal status, and baseline lipid profile? What is the effect on CHD risk of hormone replacement therapy initiated or reinstituted at various ages after menopause? How is response to diet modification affected by age, menopausal status, and hormone replacement therapy? What are the interactive effects of diet, exercise, and hormone replacement therapy on plasma lipids and CHD risk?

Future studies should be well-controlled and prospective, with care taken to control for confounding factors with clear endpoints, such as the documented training effect and decreased morbidity and mortality from CHD. For now, it appears appropriate to recommend hormone replacement therapy for many postmenopausal women, as it has been shown to decrease cardiovascular and osteoporosis risk as well as improve symptoms of estrogen deficiency. As health-care providers for women, we should be encouraging our patients to adopt a healthy lifestyle well before the climacteric, including discontinuing smoking, consuming a diet low in fat and high in complex carbohydrates, and exercising.

Note added in proof: Recently, the well-controlled, multicenter PEPI trial assessed the differences between placebo, unopposed estrogen, and each of three estrogen/progestin regimens on four endpoints related to cardiovascular risk: serum HDL, systolic blood pressure, serum insulin, and fibrinogen. It was concluded that while unopposed estrogen is optimal for HDL elevation, all hormone treatments were significantly better than placebo, and HDL averaged 2.4 mg/dl higher in women treated with the least effective of the active regimens compared with placebo. In women with a uterus, 0.625 mg/day of conjugated equine estrogens plus cyclic micronized progesterone, 200 mg/day for 12 days/month, had the most favorable effect on HDL and no excess risk of endometrial hyperplasia.

REFERENCES

1. Wenger NK, Speroff L, Packard B. Cardiovascular health and disease in women. N Engl J Med 1993; 329:247.
2. Lerner DJ, Kannel WB. Patterns of coronary heart disease morbidity and mortality in the sexes: a 26 year follow-up of Framingham population. Am Heart J 1986; 11:383–390.
3. Colditz GA, Willett WC, Stampfer MJ, et al. Menopause and the risk of coronary heart disease in women. N Engl J Med 1987; 316: 1105–1110.

4. Kris-Etherton PM, Krummel D. Role of nutrition in the prevention and treatment of coronary heart disease in women. J Am Diet Assoc 1993; 93:987–993.
5. Speroff L, Glass RH, Kase NG. Clinical Gynecologic Endocrinology and Infertility. 5th ed. Philadelphia: Williams & Wilkins, 1994.
6. Psaty B, et al. A review of the association of estrogen and progestin with cardiovascular disease in postmenopausal women. Arch Intern Med 1993; 153:1421–1427.
7. Sitruk-Ware R, Ibarra de Palacios P. Oestrogen replacement therapy and cardiovascular disease in postmenopausal women: A review. Maturitas 1989; 11:259–274.
8. Grady D, Rubin SM, Pettiti DB, et al. Hormone therapy to prevent disease and prolong life in postmenopausal women. Ann Intern Med 12; 1015–1037.
9. Pettiti DB, Perlman JA, Sidney S. Noncontraceptive estrogen and mortality: long term follow-up of women in Walnut Creek Study. Obstet Gynecol 1987; 70:289.
10. Henderson BE, Paganini-Hill A, Ross RK. Estrogen replacement therapy and protection from acute myocardial infarction. Am J Obstet Gynecol 1988; 159:312.
11. Stampfer MJ, et al. Postmenopausal estrogen therapy and cardiovascular disease: ten year follow-up from the Nurses Health Study. N Engl J Med 1991; 325:756.
12. Bush TL, Barrett-Connor E, et al. Cardiovascular mortality and noncontraceptive use of estrogen in women: results from Lipid Research Clinics Program Follow-up Study. Circulation 1987; 75: 1102.
13. Perlman J, Wolf P, et al. Menopause and the epidemiology of cardiovascular disease in women. Prog Clin Biol Res 1989; 320:283.
14. Gordon T, Kannel WB, Hjortland MC, McNamara PM. Menopause and coronary heart disease: The Framingham Study. Ann Intern Med 1978; 89:157.
15. Wilson PWF, Garrison RJ, Castelli WP. Postmenopausal estrogen use, cigarette smoking and cardiovascular morbidity in women over 50: The Framingham Study. N Engl J Med 1985; 313:1038.
16. Stevenson JC, Crook D, Godsland IF. Influence of age and menopause on serum lipids and lipoproteins in healthy women. Atherosclerosis 1993; 98:83–90.
17. Avila MH, Walker AM, Jick H. Use of replacement estrogen and risk of myocardial infarction. Epidemiology 1990; 1:128–135.

18. Shewmon DA. Lipids, atherosclerosis and postmenopausal women. Obstet Gynecol Clin North Am 1994; 21(2).

19. Soma M, et al. The lowering of lipoprotein (a) induced by estrogen plus progesterone replacement therapy in postmenopausal women. Arch Intern Med 1993; 153:1462–1468.

20. Walsh BW, et al. Effects of postmenopausal estrogen replacement on the concentration and metabolism of plasma lipoproteins. N Engl J Med 1991; 325:1196–2014.

21. Barrett-Connor E, Miller V. Estrogens, lipids and heart disease. Clin Geriatr Med 1993; 9:57.

22. Hough JL, Zilversmit DB. Effect of 17β-estradiol on aortic cholesterol content and metabolism in cholesterol-fed rabbits. Arteriosclerosis 1986; 6:57–63.

23. Hirvonen E, Malkonen M, Manninen V. Effects of different progestogens on lipoproteins during postmenopausal replacement therapy. N Engl J Med 1981; 304:560–563.

24. Sacks FM, Walsh BW. The effects of reproductive hormones on serum lipoproteins: unresolved issues in biology and clinical practice. Ann NY Acad Sci 1990; 592:272–285, 334–345.

25. Tikkanen MJ, Kuusi T, et al. Postmenopausal hormone replacement therapy: effects of progestogens on serum lipids and lipoproteins: A review. Maturitas 1986; 8:7–17.

26. Barrett-Connor E, Wingard DL, Criqui MH. Postmenopausal estrogen use and heart disease risk factors in the 1980's. JAMA 1989; 261:2095–2100.

27. Nabulsi AA, et al. (ARIC). Association of hormone replacement therapy with various cardiovascular risk factors in postmenopausal women. N Engl J Med 1993; 328:1069–1075.

28. Hegele RA. Lipoprotein (a): an emerging risk factor for atherosclerosis. Can J Cardiol 1989; 5:263–265.

29. Gambrell RD, Teran AZ. Changes in lipid and lipoprotein with long term estrogen deficiency and hormone replacement therapy. Am J Obstet Gynecol 1991; 165:307–317.

30. Weinstein L, Bewtra C, Gallagher JC. Evaluation of a continuous combined low-dose regimen of estrogen-progestin for treatment of the menopausal patient. Am J Obstet Gynecol 1990; 162:1534–1542.

31. Christiansen C, Riis BJ. Five years with continued combined oestrogen/progestogen therapy. Effects on calcium metabolism, lipoproteins and bleeding pattern. Br J Obstet Gynaecol 1990; 97:1087–1092.

32. Sigmund W, Becker DM. The Johns Hopkins Physicians Lipid Education Program. Baltimore: Johns Hopkins University Press, 1988:35.
33. Kris-Etherton PM, et al. The effect of diet on plasma lipids, lipoproteins and coronary heart disease: National Cholesterol Education Program. J Am Diet Assoc 1988; 88:1373.
34. Mensink RP, Katan MB. Effect of a diet enriched with monounsaturated or polyunsaturated fatty acids on levels of low-density lipoprotein and high-density lipoprotein cholesterol in healthy women and men. N Engl J Med 1989; 321:436–441.
35. Grundy SM, Denke MA. Dietary influences on serum lipids and lipoproteins. J Lipid Res 1990; 31:1149–1172.
36. Mata P, et al. Effect of dietary monounsaturated fatty acids on plasma lipoproteins and apolipoproteins in women. Am J Clin Nutr 1992; 56:77–83.
37. Stampfer MJ, et al. Vitamin E consumption and the risk of coronary heart disease in women. N Engl J Med 1993; 328:1444–1449.
38. Smith-Schneider LM, Sigman-Grant MJ, Kris-Etherton PM. Dietary fat reduction strategies. J Am Diet Assoc 1992; 92:34–38.
39. Dattilo AM, Kris-Etherton PM. Effects of weight reduction on blood lipids and lipoproteins: a meta-analysis. Am J Clin Nutr 1992; 56:320–328.
40. Andersson B, Seidell J, Terning K, Bjorntorp B. Influence of menopause on dietary treatment of obesity. J Intern Med 1990; 227: 173–181.
41. Taylor PA, Ward AM. Women, high-density lipoprotein cholesterol and exercise. Arch Intern Med 1993; 153:1178–1184.
42. Svendsen O, Hassager C, Christiansen C. Effect of an energy-restrictive diet, with or without exercise, on lean tissue mass, resting metabolic rate, cardiovascular risk factors and bone in overweight postmenopausal women. Am J Med 1993; 95:131–140.
43. Nieman DC, et al. Reducing-diet and exercise-training effects on serum lipids and lipoproteins in mildly obese women. Am J Clin Nutr 1990; 52:640–645.
44. The Writing Group for the PEPI Trial. Effects of estrogen/progestin regimens on heart disease risk factors in postmenopausal women. JAMA 1995; 273:199–208.

9

The Role of Exercise in Reducing Cardiovascular Risk After the Menopause

Kelly Anne Spratt and Eric L. Michelson

Medical College of Pennsylvania
and Hahnemann University
Philadelphia, Pennsylvania

A body in motion tends to stay in motion, a body at rest tends to stay at rest.

Isaac Newton (1)

I. OVERVIEW

The female half of the demographic swell known as the baby boomers is now approaching menopause, and they have applied the same characteristic "take-charge" philosophy to this phase of their lives that has marked every other. By the year 2000, it is expected that nearly 700 million women worldwide will be over the age of 50 years. In the United States alone, 38% of all women will be over the age of 45 years (2). By and large, however, the vast majority of these women are sedentary. Several population studies note that less than 25% of women regularly exercise (3). It is likely that even fewer postmenopausal women are engaged in regular vigorous activity. One recent report estimated that physical inactivity accounts for approximately 25% of all chronic diseases in the United States (4). Since cardiovascular disease remains the leading cause of mortality and morbidity for women in this age group, a preventive strategy focused on cardiovascular risk-factor modification will continue to be the cornerstone for maintaining high quality of life during this period. This chapter focuses on the beneficial aspects of exercise in reducing the risk of cardiovascular disease in postmenopausal women.

In the premenopausal years, women seem to be protected from development of coronary artery disease compared to their male counterparts. This observation has led to the erroneous conclusion that coronary artery disease is a "male" disease. The loss of estrogen at the time of the menopause is associated with a marked increase in the manifestations of coronary disease in women (5,6). Data associating a decline in estrogen with an unfavorable lipid profile similar to that of men has been believed to be the mechanism for this dramatic increase in coronary disease (7,8). However, additional evidence is now available that demonstrates the potential importance of direct vasodilating and other properties of estrogen (9–12).

Exercise has been believed to attenuate the unfavorable lipid changes associated with the onset of menopause, which include elevation of serum total cholesterol, low-density lipoprotein (LDL) cholesterol, and triglycerides, and decline in high-density lipoprotein (HDL) cholesterol. In addition, exercise promotes beneficial hemodynamic changes that mitigate the initiation and progression of coronary artery disease by modification of cardiovascular risk factors such as hypertension, diabetes mellitus, and obesity. Finally, regular exercise tends to promote healthy behaviors such as smoking cessation, feelings of well-being, and social interaction, which are currently under evaluation for their positive impact on cardiovascular health. In this chapter, these metabolic, hemodynamic, and psychosocial benefits of exercise for postmenopausal women are discussed, and strategies for successfully incorporating exercise into a comprehensive program of cardiovascular risk-factor modification are addressed.

II. WHAT IS EXERCISE?

Although there is much evidence that physically active persons have decreased morbidity when compared with sedentary persons, exactly what qualifies as exercise is still debated. Defining this term is especially important for women who may be engaged in vigorous homemaking activity that could qualify as exercise. Recently, the energy expenditure of several homemaking tasks was evaluated in women known to have coronary artery disease. (13). These tasks involve mild to moderate levels of energy expenditure and, if completed serially, may be a valuable source of exercise, especially for older women. Women have been excluded from most of the larger studies on physical activity and physical fitness. The data available on men may or may not apply to the same degree to women, although the trend would indicate, from those studies in which women have been included, that exercise is beneficial.

The Harvard Alumni Study used two questionnaires administered in 1962 or 1966 and then again in 1977 to assess physi-

cal activity of the 10,269 men in the study (14). The respondents
reported daily number of city blocks walked and stairs climbed,
and type, frequency, and duration of participation in sports or
recreational activities in hours per week. Each activity was assigned a value of kilocalories, and sports activity was assessed
according to metabolic equivalents (METs). One MET—the energy expended per minute while sitting quietly—is equivalent to
3.5 ml of oxygen uptake per kg of body weight per minute for an
adult weighing 70 kg. Light sports activity was defined as that
requiring less than 4.5 METs, while moderate vigorous activity
required more than 4.5 METs. The most common moderate vigorous activities included swimming, tennis, jogging, and running. The total activity performed generated a physical activity
index that divided the group into quartiles. In these men, moderately vigorous activity greater than 2000 kcal/week was associated with a 23% lower risk of death due to cardiovascular disease
than in the least active quartile (14). In a recent follow-up of this
cohort, a graded inverse relationship between total physical activity and mortality was reported (15).

Another group of authors used a cycle ergometer to define a
measurable workload assessing levels of fitness rather than simply activity in 1960 men and quantitated decreased risk from
cardiovascular disease (16). Again, the most fit group had less
than half the cardiovascular mortality of the least fit group.

The Framingham Heart Study released data on 1404 women
correlating physical activity and mortality (17). The assessment of
physical activity did not use a formally validated questionnaire
to assess activity and did not include additional information on
level of fitness. The women were asked how much time they
spent sleeping, resting, and performing light, moderate, or heavy
activity on a daily basis. Use of such surveys to document physical activity could introduce a certain degree of inaccuracy because patients decide what constitutes "light" or "heavy." The
authors concluded that there was no difference in cardiovascular
mortality and activity between active and sedentary women.
Active women did appear to live longer, but this benefit was
attributed to a decrease in cancer deaths.

It becomes evident that, when prescribing activity for our patients with prevention of cardiovascular mortality as the goal, it is necessary to specify activity of a particular intensity and duration. Both the intensity and the duration of activity needed to improve physical conditioning, achieve physical fitness, and maximize cardiovascular protection vary among individuals. Although there appears to be a linear relationship between intensity of exercise and cardioprotection, substantial benefit is seen with mild to moderate exercise, especially in previously sedentary women. The American Heart Association guidelines (18) for exercise standards suggest that as little as 20 minutes of walking vigorously three times per week or, at a more moderate pace, 30 minutes five times per week can provide cardioprotection. The minimum amount of weekly activity for all persons is 700 kilocalories (about 6–7 miles). The Harvard Alumni Study suggests that maximal cardioprotective effect is seen with exercise activity that exceeds 2000 kilocalories weekly (walking 20 miles per week) (14) and that vigorous activity (greater than 6 METs) promotes longevity in middle-aged men (15). However, the AHA guidelines emphasize that exercise need not be of high intensity to be beneficial. Mild to moderate activity performed for a longer duration is cardioprotective, and often associated with fewer orthopedic injuries. This is an important factor for postmenopausal women, who may be susceptible to osteoporotic fractures. In this population, exercise of mild to moderate intensity, approximately 3–6 METs three to five times weekly, appears to safely achieve cardioprotection and ensure long-term participation. It is also important to emphasize to older, somewhat more frail, women that daily household tasks may also serve as a source of mild, yet still beneficial, exercise. The METs of common activities are listed in Table 1.

III. EFFECT OF EXERCISE ON LIPIDS

The lipid profile of a postmenopausal woman demonstrates an increase in atherogenic risk factors such as lower HDL choles-

Table 1 Metabolic Equivalents
(METs) of Common Activities

Activity	METs
Baking	2.0
Dancing	
Ballroom	2.9
Square	5.5
Aerobic	6.0
Golf	
With cart	2.5
Without cart	4.9
Walking	
2.0 miles per hour	2.5
4.0 miles per hour	4.5
Gardening	4.4
Swimming	
Slow	4.5
Fast	7.0
Badminton	5.5
Roller skating	6.5
Tennis (doubles)	6.0
Washing dishes	2.0
Vacuuming carpet	3.0
Changing bed	3.6
Washing floor	4.0
Sexual intercourse	2.0–4.0

terol and increased levels of serum triglycerides, total cholesterol, LDL cholesterol, and apolipoproteins A1 and B. Abnormal lipid profiles represent a combination of genetic predisposing derangements and factors affected by diet, age, weight, hormonal status, medications, and exercise. Data on the beneficial effects of lipid reduction in at-risk individuals are now convincing, and medications such as hydroxymethylglutaryl coenzyme A (HMG-CoA) reductase inhibitors should be a mainstay of therapy (19). While the role of exercise in lowering lipids is more modest, it is certainly not insignificant. Despite this, most studies on the beneficial effects of exercise on lipids and coronary artery disease have included either predominantly or exclusively men. In an overview of all observational studies of exercise and cardio-vascular disease, only five of 43 studies included or reported data on women (20). Thus, few studies have unequivocally docu-mented the benefit of exercise on these lipid abnormalities in women in general and postmenopausal women in particular. In addition, confounding variables such as fluctuating hormonal status, intensity, duration and type of exercise, and smoking status have contributed to a lack of consensus and dearth of documentation on the effect of exercise on lipids in postmeno-pausal women.

Given that less conclusive data on postmenopausal women are available, one option would be extrapolation of the extensive data on the beneficial effect of exercise on lipids that have been collected on men. A recent evaluation of 458 men and women enrolled in cardiac rehabilitation and exercise training illustrated that the changes in lipids were similar in both sexes but reached statistical significance only in men due to the larger number of men ($n = 375$) than women ($n = 83$) in the study (21). Both men and women enrolled in the 12-week phase II cardiac rehabilitation/exercise program experienced similar percentages of decline in serum total cholesterol and triglycerides and increases in HDL cholesterol. Given that many of the studies of exercise have underrepresented women, one could postulate that any lack of clear-cut positive cardiovascular impact could be due to the in-adequate number of female patients.

A major mechanism by which regular exercise may exert a beneficial effect on cardiovascular risk is modulation of circulat-ing lipoproteins. For example, lipoprotein lipase facilitates clear-ance of circulating triglycerides. The acute phase of exercise increases levels of lipoprotein lipase in both adipose and muscle tissue (22). With endurance training, there is an increase in the muscle microvasculature. Since lipoprotein lipase is associated with capillary endothelium, this increase in capillaries also con-tributes to an increase in lipoprotein lipase, which has been documented in trained endurance athletes (23). The lower tri-glyceride levels seen in women who are regular exercisers may be due in part to this phenomenon. Recent studies have demonstrated that elevated triglyceride levels are associated with markedly increased cardiovascular risk for women (24). Lipoprotein lipase is also directly related to HDL cholesterol such that increases in lipoprotein lipase augment HDL cholesterol levels (25). The response of HDL cholesterol to exercise in women is not clearly defined. Although some cross-sectional studies have noted higher levels of HDL in regular exercisers compared to sedentary persons, most interventional studies that have included women have noted minimal change in HDL cholesterol levels (26). However, one study that included subfractionation of HDL cholesterol demonstrated a shift, over a period of 12 weeks, in quantity of HDL-3 to the apparently more cardioprotective HDL-2 (27). In premenopausal women, HDL-2 predominates; however, at the onset of menopause, the level of HDL-3 begins to rise. Hepatic lipase is the enzyme that catalyzes the conversion of HDL-2 to the less cardioprotective HDL-3, and exercise appears to inhibit this enzyme. Thus, while total levels of HDL cholesterol may appear to remain similar, it may be speculated that cardioprotection is augmented with exercise.

On the other hand, an increase in total HDL cholesterol levels has been shown to occur with fairly strenuous exercise over a prolonged period of time. However, in one study of 22 women, as their weekly running mileage was increased vigorously from 3.5 to 45 miles, their mean HDL cholesterol levels increased relatively modestly, from 53 to 58 mg/dl (28). The challenge of recommending activity of this intensity as a general exercise prescription for the vast majority of postmenopausal women would be daunting to female patients and health care providers alike. The probable cardioprotective benefits of changes in the subfractions of HDL cholesterol that may be achieved with more moderate levels of exercise over a period as brief as 12 weeks is more readily implemented, especially in women who may be undertaking an exercise program for the first time.

Circulating apolipoproteins such as A-1 and B have been shown to correlate strongly with risk for coronary artery disease. Apolipoprotein A-1 is associated with HDL cholesterol and is considered cardiprotective, while elevated apolipoprotein B or a low apolipoprotein A-1/B ratio confers an increased risk for atherosclerotic cardiovascular disease. Cross-sectional studies of exercising females demonstrate lower levels of apolipoprotein B and higher apolipoprotein A-1/B ratios (27,29). In a smaller cohort of women with an additional risk factor for coronary artery disease—cigarette smoking—those women who exercised had lower apolipoprotein B levels and a higher apolipoprotein A-1/B ratio (30).

Exercise has minimal impact on LDL cholesterol levels, although a few studies have demonstrated a slight decrease in LDL cholesterol levels with regular exercise. However, LDL cholesterol, like HDL cholesterol, has subfractions of which the cardiovascular impact has yet to be completely defined. In further studies of the impact of exercise on lipids, inclusion of these subtypes of LDL cholesterol could be considered.

IV. EFFECT OF EXERCISE ON BLOOD PRESSURE

The incidence of both systolic and diastolic hypertension increases with age. This marked increase in the number of women developing hypertension during the menopause not only increases cardiovascular vulnerability for women but also represents a major public health issue with respect to health care resources. Measures to maintain normotension include diet, hormone replacement therapy, weight control, smoking cessation, and exercise. Even modest reductions in blood pressure can substantially reduce mortality and morbidity from hypertensive cardiovascular and cerebrovascular disease, as well as from other target-organ disease.

The reasons for the apparent increase in hypertension with menopause is likely multifactorial. Estrogen appears to influence the blood-pressure response to mental stressors more than to physical stressors. In a recent study, ambulatory cardiovascular monitoring and serum norepinephrine levels were obtained to evaluate responses to both mental and physical stressors. Heart rate, blood pressure, and norepinephrine levels inversely correlated with serum estradiol levels (31). These augmented responses especially increase cardiovascular morbidity and mortality in postmenopausal women with coronary artery disease. Hypertension also contributes to left ventricular hypertrophy, which independently increases risk for development of cardiovascular events.

Dynamic exercise results in vasodilation in skeletal muscle and capillary proliferation, both of which decrease systemic peripheral resistance and ultimately lead to a decrease in systolic and diastolic blood pressure. Exercise is effective in reducing blood pressure in both normotensive and hypertensive patients, so clinicians may comfortably advise that it is still beneficial to begin an exercise program even after the onset of hypertension. The Hypertension and Ambulatory Recording Venetia Study (HARVEST) Group recently reported the effect of moderate exercise on stage I hypertension (systolic blood pressure 140–159 mm Hg and diastolic blood pressure 90–99 mm Hg) (32). Although the difference in systolic blood pressure was not statistically different, regular exercisers demonstrated significant decreases in diastolic blood pressure. This study also noted that the resting heart rate and urinary norepinephrine levels were lower in exercisers than in their sedentary counterparts. The authors suggest that sympathetic withdrawal is an important mechanism by which exercise decreases blood pressure. Among exercisers, no incremental benefit was noted between subjects participating in strenuous competitive sports and those who engaged in more moderate activity. In this group of young (less than 45 years old) patients, no benefit on blood pressure was noted when patients participated in light activity such as walking or gardening versus those patients who were sedentary. However, others have noted that, in elderly female patients who may be completely sedentary, a program of light physical activity may be beneficial (33).

A recent compilation of several studies of the effect of moderate exercise on blood pressure indicates that regular exercise could decrease blood pressure by an average of 13 mm Hg systolic and 10 mm Hg diastolic (34). Given the prevalence of hypertension among postmenopausal women and the morbidity associated with this disease, such a decrease in blood pressure could have a tremendously favorable impact on health care outcomes and decreased utilization of resources to treat target-organ disease.

V. EFFECT OF EXERCISE ON OBESITY

One of the major benefits of exercise appears to be a decrease in both total body weight and composition of body fat. A gradual increase in weight through the adult years is usual, and the effect of menopause on this weight gain has not been completely defined. In 541 women aged 42–50 years studied over a 3-year period, an average weight gain of 2.25 kg was noted (35). Although the range of weight change varied from a loss of 14 kg to a gain of 32 kg, over 20% of the women gained 4.5 kg or more. A 1990 change in the United States weight guidelines for women older than 35 years greatly increased the upper limit of desirable body mass index (36). However, more recent data suggest that, for middle-aged women, even weight in the "normal" range increases the risk of coronary heart disease and the current weight guidelines are falsely reassuring to a large number of middle-aged women (37).

Women are especially vulnerable to the detrimental effects of obesity on the cardiovascular risk profile (24). For this group of at-risk women, exercise is a low-risk, low-cost means of maintaining a lower body weight. In a group of 458 patients enrolled in a phase II cardiac rehabilitation program (average age 63 years), both men and women had a statistically significant decrease in body fat (21). Among elderly women (age >70 years), those who participated in moderate activity had a significant decrease in both body mass index and weight compared to those who were completely sedentary (38). No further decrease in weight was noted as the level of exercise was increased from the intermediate level to most active level. Active women tend to have a lower overall body weight with a decreased percentage of body fat. In addition, evaluation of the dietary patterns of active women reveals a similar caloric intake but a greater percentage of carbohydrate and a smaller percentage of fat intake compared to those of their sedentary peers (30). The effect of this dietary modification, when reinforced by regular exercise, appears to contribute to longer-term control of obesity and overall general cardiovascular health.

The adverse effects of weight gain on the cardiovascular risk profile may be due in part to the distribution of the body fat, with truncal or intraabdominal body fat portending a greater risk of cardiovascular disease (39,40). Aerobic exercise promotes the loss of abdominal fat more readily than fat at any other site (41). Increased abdominal obesity is associated with increased cardiovascular risk by several potential mechanisms. In particular, truncal obesity is associated with alteration of carbohydrate metabolism, resulting in decreased insulin receptor sensitivity, increased levels of plasma insulin (hyperinsulinemia), and decreased glucose tolerance. Insulin enhances proliferation of arterial smooth-muscle cells and formation of lipid deposits in arterial walls. Hyperinsulinemia significantly increases risk of development of coronary artery disease. However, even normal-weight postmenopausal women demonstrate mild hyperinsulinemia, which may be related to loss of estrogen (42). The preferential reduction of truncal obesity with aerobic exercise mitigates this hyperinsulinemia. In addition, muscle-strengthening exercises decrease insulin resistance in skeletal muscle and ultimately results in lower fasting insulin levels. Even a single bout of submaximal exercise enhances insulin sensitivity in skeletal muscle, a benefit that may persist for hours or even days. In a study of postmenopausal women exercising three times per week at 70–85% of maximal heart rate on either treadmill or resistive training equipment, both groups had improved glucose tolerance and insulin response compared to controls (43). Thus, both aerobic and muscle-strengthening exercises are beneficial in reducing hyperinsulinemia. Women are more likely to develop diabetes than men, and both insulin- and noninsulin-dependent diabetic women should be strongly encourage to begin an exercise regimen to decrease fasting plasma glucose and insulin levels and mitigate diabetic end-organ complications.

VI. EFFECT OF EXERCISE ON THE FIBRINOLYTIC SYSTEM

The elevated cardiovascular risk that has been noted with increased levels of fibrinogen has been well documented (44,45). In the Postmenopausal Estrogen/Progestin Intervention Trial, postmenopausal women given placebo had an increase in fibrinogen levels (46). This is suggestive that with the onset of menopause fibrinogen levels increase, representing an additional source of cardiovascular risk during this period. Persons who regularly perform moderate to vigorous exercise have been noted to have decreased levels of fibrinogen (30,47). Additionally, acute exercise has been noted to potentiate fibrinolytic activity due to increased release of plasminogen activator from vascular endothelium, enhanced prostacyclin activity, and increased inhibitory capacity of antithrombin III (48). In sedentary men who began a moderate exercise program, platelet adhesiveness and aggregation were depressed while more strenuous exercise had the opposite effect (49). The effects of various degrees of exercise on hemostatic factors need to be further addressed, especially in postmenopausal women.

VII. EFFECT OF EXERCISE ON ARRHYTHMIAS

Atrial and ventricular arrhythmias increase with age and thus represent an important source of potential morbidity for aging, postmenopausal women. In some patients, exercise may provoke intolerable arrhythmias that require directed therapy and limitation of exercise until controlled. In most patients, however, arrhythmias do not limit moderate activity. Animal studies have demonstrated that regular exercise promotes cardiac electrical stability and increases the ventricular fibrillation threshold even during hypoxia and acute myocardial ischemia (50). Regular exercise attenuates sympathetic activity and augments vago-mimetic responsiveness, suggesting that catecholamine-mediated arrhythmias might decrease with regular exercise. Decreases in catecholamine levels often persist throughout the day with train-ing, and may provide substantial benefit with respect to risk for ischemic events, vascular occlusive phenomena, and sudden car-diac death. One group evaluated 184 healthy older persons (mean age 68 years; 43% men, 57% women) to determine if moderate exercise, short- or long-term, prolongs time to cardiovascular events in older persons. In 2 years of follow-up, 2.4% of the exercisers experienced a new cardiovascular event while 12.9% of the controls had a new event. The most common new cardio-vascular event in the controls was an arrhythmia, and the authors postulate that a major cardioprotective effect of exercise is against development of clinically significant arrhythmias (51).

VIII.   EXERCISE IN CARDIAC REHABILITATION: THE NEED FOR SECONDARY PREVENTION

Cardiovascular disease, when manifest in women, is associated with a higher mortality and morbidity than in men, which is at least in part due to the older age of the patient at the time of onset and more comorbidities. Prescription of exercise as part of a complete cardiac rehabilitation program is associated with a de-crease in subsequent cardiovascular mortality of 20–30%. Al-though part of this decrease may be attributed to reduction of other cardiovascular risk factors, exercise itself has positive he-modynamic effects on the cardiovascular system. The neuro-humoral benefits of a training program following myocardial infarction has been shown in an early report of small group of patients enrolled in the Exercise in Anterior Myocardial Infarc-tion (EAMI) trial. Preliminary data suggest that 6 months of a training program normalized heart-rate variability in patients with previously documented decreased heart-rate variability

(52). Decreased heart-rate variability has been shown to be a harbinger of a worse outcome following myocardial infarction (53). It is thus particularly disconcerting that fewer women are offered the option of cardiac rehabilitation, and, when offered, women drop out of rehabilitation more frequently and sooner than their male counterparts. One meta-analysis of over 4500 cardiac rehabilitation patients notes that only 3% of the patients were women (54).

The etiology for this low participation in cardiac rehabilitation is likely multifactorial and may include the older age and increased comorbidities of female patients, less experience and familiarity with exercise and exercise equipment, and the perceived time-consuming responsibility of female patients to care for other members of their family. Even the greater rate of depression after myocardial infarction seen in women with cardiovascular disease (55) may contribute to this lower desire to participate in exercise programs.

IX. EXERCISE IN THE MANAGEMENT OF CONGESTIVE HEART FAILURE

Women with congestive heart failure also appear to benefit from exercise training and cardiac rehabilitation. The marked fatigue and exercise intolerance experienced by patients with congestive heart failure may be due, at least in part, to skeletal muscle and neurohumoral aberrations. Skeletal muscles of these patients demonstrate atrophy, abnormal blood flow, and histological changes, each of which contributes to poor exercise capacity (56). Regular exercise training in this group of patients has been shown to increase exercise capacity, decrease symptoms of dyspnea, and improve daily-activity scores (57). In addition, regular exercise decreases plasma catecholamine levels and enhances heart-rate variability (57). Each of these changes may be associated with an improvement in the long-term prognosis in patients with congestive heart failure. A subset of the Studies of Left Ventricular Dysfunction (SOLVD) Trial documented that patients with an improved 6-minute walk test (a measure of exercise capacity) had a lower overall morbidity and mortality (58). However, extensive long-term data on the impact of exercise on mortality in patients with congestive heart failure are not yet available. The current evidence does suggest that this is an important modality to improve functional capacity and quality of life, and should be encouraged as part of a monitored cardiac rehabilitation program.

Despite the low number of female patients in cardiac rehabilitation exercise programs, women with ischemic heart disease would seem to benefit from prescribed, monitored exercise—at least to an extent similar to that for men. Further emphasis on participation in exercise as part of a comprehensive secondary prevention strategy is indicated.

X. FUTURE DIRECTIONS

Future research on the benefits of prescribed exercise in older women is warranted to optimize benefit, encourage participation, and document cost-effectiveness. Exercise must be viewed as an accessible, low-cost, low-risk intervention for improving total health, wellness, longevity, and cardiovascular function, and as a primary preventive strategy for reducing cardiovascular risk. This approach is particularly relevant to the care of postmenopausal women. Physicians should be encouraged to include exercise prescriptions in their patient-management plans.

REFERENCES

1. Adapted from Newton's Laws of Motion. In: Ballentyne DWG, Walker LEQ. A Dictionary of Named Effects and Laws. London: Chapman and Hall, 1961.
2. US Senate Special Committee on Aging. Aging America: Trends and Projections. Washington, DC: United States Department of Health and Human Services, 1988.
3. Prevalence of recommended levels of physical activity among

women—Behavioral Risk Factor Surveillance System, 1992. J Am Med Assoc 1995; 273:986–987.

4. McGinnis JM, Foege WH. Actual causes of death in the United States. J Am Med Assoc 1993; 270:2207–2212.

5. Matthews KA, Meilahn E, Kuller LH, Kelsey SF, Caggiula AW, Wing RR. Menopause and risk factors for coronary heart disease. N Engl J Med 1989; 321:641–646.

6. Gordon T, Kannel WB, Hjortland MC, McNamara PM. Menopause and coronary heart disease: the Framingham study. Ann Intern Med 1978; 89:157–161.

7. Stevenson JC, Crook D, Godsland IF. Influence of age and menopause on serum lipids and lipoproteins in healthy women. Arteriosclerosis 1993; 98:89–90.

8. Razay G, Heaton KW, Bolton CH. Coronary heart disease risk factors in relation to the menopause. Q J Med 1992; 85:889–896.

9. Reis SE, Gloth ST, Blumenthal RS, Resar JR, Zacur HA, Gerstenblith G, Brinker JA. Ethinyl estradiol acutely attenuates abnormal coronary vasomotor responses to acetylcholine in postmenopausal women. Circulation 1994; 89:52–60.

10. Leiberman EH, Gerhard MD, Uehata A, Walsh BW, Selwyn AP, Ganz P, Yeung AC, Creager MA. Estrogen improves endothelium-derived, flow-mediated vasodilation in postmenopausal women. Ann Intern Med 1994; 121:936–941.

11. Williams JK, Adams MR, Herrington DM, Clarkson TB. Short-term administration of estrogen and vascular responses of atherosclerotic coronary arteries. J Am Coll Cardiol 1992; 20:452–457.

12. Gilligan DM, Badar DM, Panza JA, Quyyumi AA, Cannon RO. Effects of estrogen replacement therapy on peripheral vasomotor function in postmenopausal women. Am J Cardiol 1995; 75: 264–268.

13. Wilke NA, Sheldahl LM, Dougherty SM, Hanna RD, Nickele GA, Tristani FE. Energy expenditure during household tasks in women with coronary artery disease. Am J Cardiol 1995; 75:670–674.

14. Paffenbarger RS, Hyse PH, Wing AL, Lee IM, Jung DL, Kampert JB. The association of changes in physical activity level and other lifestyle characteristics with mortality among men. N Engl J Med 1993; 328:538–545.

15. Lee I-M, Hsieh CC, Paffenbarger RS. Exercise intensity and longevity in men: The Harvard Alumni Study. J Am Med Assoc 1995; 273:1179–1184.

16. Sandvik L, Erikkssen J, Thaulow E, Erikssen G, Mundal R, Rodahl K. Physical fitness as a predictor of mortality among healthy, middle-aged men. N Engl J Med 1993; 328:533–537.
17. Sherman SE, D'Agostino RB, Cobb JL, Kannel WB. Physical activity and mortality in women in the Framingham Heart Study. Am Heart J 1994; 128:879–884.
18. Fletcher GF, Balady G, Froelicher VF, Hartley LH, Haskell WL, Pollock ML. American Heart Association Medical/Scientific Statement. Exercise standards: A statement for healthcare professionals from the American Heart Association. Circulation 1995; 91:580–615.
19. Scandinavian Simvastatin Survival Study Group. Randomised trial of cholesterol lowering in 4444 patients with coronary heart disease: the Scandinavian Simvastatin Survival Study (4S). Lancet 1994; 344:1383–1389.
20. Powell KE, Thompson PD, Caspersen CJ, Kendrick JS. Physical activity and the incidence of coronary heart disease. Annu Rev Public Health 1989; 8:253–287.
21. Lavie CJ, Milani RV. Effects of cardiac rehabilitation and exercise training on exercise capacity, coronary risk factors, behavioral characteristics, and quality of life in women. Am J Cardiol 1995; 75: 340–343.
22. MacCauley D. Exercise, cardiovascular disease and lipids. Br J Clin Pract 1993; 47:323–327.
23. Nikkila EA, Taskinen MP, Rehunen S, Harkonen M. Lipoprotein lipase activity in adipose tissue and skeletal muscle of runners: relation to serum lipoproteins. Metabolism 1978; 27:1661–1671.
24. Bengtsson C, Bjorkelund, Lapidus L, Lissner L. Associations of serum lipid concentrations and obesity with mortality in women: 20 year follow up of participants in prospective population study in Gothenburg, Sweden. Br Med J 1993; 307:1385–1388.
25. MacAuley D. Exercise, cardiovascular disease and lipids. Br J Clin Prac 1993; 47:323–327.
26. Taylor PA, Ward A. Women, high-density lipoprotein cholesterol and exercise. Arch Intern Med 1993; 153:1178–1184.
27. Blumenthal JA, Matthews K, Fredrikson M, Rifai N, Schniebolk S, German D, Stiege J, Rodin J. Effects of exercise training on cardiovascular function and plasma lipid, lipoprotein and apolipoprotein concentrations in premenopausal and postmenopausal women. Arterioscler Thromb 1991; 11:912–917.
28. Rotkis T, Boyden W, Parmenter RW, Stanforth P, Wilmore J. High

density lipoprotein cholesterol and body composition of female runners. Metabolism 1981; 30:994–995.

29. Lamon-Fava S, Fisher EC, Nelson ME, Evans WJ, Millar JS, Ordovas JM, Schaefer EJ. Effect of exercise and menstrual cycle status on plasma lipids, LDL particle size and apolipoproteins. J Clin Endocrinol Metab 1989; 68:17–21.

30. Casazza GA, Holly RG, Alstini AV, Amsterdam EA. Exercise training and reduction of some coronary risk factors in female cigarette smokers. Am J Cardiol 1995; 75:85–87.

31. Owens JF, Stoney CM, Matthews KA. Menopausal status influences ambulatory blood pressure levels and blood pressure changes during mental stress. Circulation 1993; 88:2794–2802.

32. Palatini P, Graniero GR, Mormino P, Nicolosi L, Mos L, et al. Relation between physical training and ambulatory blood pressure in stage I hyertensive subjects: Results of the HARVEST trial. Circulation 1994; 90:2870–2876.

33. Reaven PD, Barrett-Connor E, Edelstein S. Relation between leisure-time activity and blood pressure in older women. Circulation 1991; 83:559–565.

34. Fentem PH. Exercise in prevention of disease. Br Med Bull 1992; 48:630–650.

35. Ring RR, Matthews KA, Kuller LH, Meilahn EN, Plantings PL. Weight gain at the time of menopause. Arch Intern Med 1991; 151: 97–102.

36. US Department of Agriculture, US Department of Health and Human Services. Nutrition and Your Health: Dietary Guidelines for Americans. 3rd ed. Washington, DC: US Government Printing Office, 1990.

37. Willett WC, Manson JE, Stampfer MJ, Colditz GA, Rosner B, Speizer FE, Hennekens CH. Weight, weight change, and coronary heart disease in women. J Am Med Assoc 1995; 273:461–465.

38. Voorrips LE, Lemmink KAPM, Van Heuvelen JG, Bult P, Van Staveren WA. The physical condition of elderly women differing in habitual physical activity. Med Sci Sports Exerc 1993; 25:1152–1157.

39. Peiris AN, Sothman MS, Hoffman RG, Hennes MI, Wilson CR, Gustafson AB, Kissenbah AH. Adiposity, fat distribution, and cardiovascular risk. Ann Intern Med 1989; 110:867–872.

40. Larsson B, Svardsudd K, Welin L, Wilhelmsen L, Bjorntorp P, Tibblin G. Abdominal adipose tissue distribution, obesity, and risk

of cardiovascular disease and death: 13 year follow up of participants in the study of men in 1913. Br Med J 1984; 288:1401–1404.

41. Despres JP, Tremblay A, Nadeau A, Bouchard C. Physical training
     and changes in regional adipose tissue distribution. Acta Med
     Scand 1988; 723(suppl):205–212.

42. Proudler AJ, Felton CV, Stevenson JC. Aging and the response of
     plasma insulin, glucose and C-peptide concentrations to intra-
     venous glucose in postmenopausal women. Clin Sci 1992; 83:
     489–494.

43. VanDam S, Gillespy M, Notelovitz M, Martin AD. Effect of exer-
     cise on glucose metabolism in postmenopausal women. Am J
     Obstet Gynecol 1988; 159:82–86.

44. Thompson SG, Kienast J, Pyke SDM, Haverkate F, van de Loo JCW.
     Hemostatic factors and the risk of myocardial infarction or sudden
     death in patients with angina pectoris. N Engl J Med 1995; 332:
     635–641.

45. Ernst E, Resch KL. Fibrinogen as a cardiovascular risk factor: a
     meta-analysis and review of the literature. Ann Intern Med 1993;
     118:956–963.

46. Writing Group for the Postmenopausal Estrogen/Progestin Inter-
     ventions Trial. Effects of Estrogen or Estrogen/Progestin Regi-
     mens of Heart Disease Risk Factors in Postmenopausal Women. J
     Am Med Assoc 1995; 273:199–208.

47. Connelly JB, Cooper JA, Meade TW. Strenuous exercise, plasma
     fibrinogen and Factor VII activity. Br Heart J 1992; 67:351–354.

48. Drygas WK. Changes in blood platelet function, coagulation and
     fibrinolytic activity in response to moderate, exhaustive and pro-
     longed activity. Int J Sports Med 1988; 9:67–72.

49. Wang J, Jen CJ, Kung H, Lin LJ, Hsiue TR, Chen H. Different effects
     of strenous exercise and moderate exercise on platelet function.
     Circulation 1994; 90:2877–2885.

50. Posel D, Noakes T, Kantor P, Lambert M, Opie LH. Exercise train-
     ing after experimental myocardial infarction increases the ven-
     tricular fibrillation threshold before and after the onset of reinfarc-
     tion in the isolated rat heart. Circulation 1989; 80:138–145.

51. Posner JD, Gorman KM, Gitlin LN, Sands LP, Kleban M, Windsor
     L, Shaw C. Effects of exercise training in the elderly and time to
     onset of cardiovascular diseases. J Am Ger Soc 1990; 38:205–210.

52. Mazzuero G, Lanfranchi P, Temporelli PL, Giannuzzi P, Colombo
     R. Influence of long-term physical training on depressed heart rate
     variability after myocardial infarction. Circulation 1994; 90:I-162.

53. Kleiger RE, Miller JP, Bigger JT, Moss AJ, and the Multicenter Post-Infarction Research Group. Decreased heart rate variability and its association with increased mortality after acute myocardial infarction. Am J Cardiol 1987; 59:256–262.
54. O'Connor GT, Buring JE, Yusuf S, Goldhaber SZ, Olmstead EM, Paffenbarger RS Jr, Hennekens CH. An overview of randomized trials of rehabilitation with exercise after myocardial infarction. Circulation 1989; 80:234–244.
55. Frasure-Smith N, Lesperance F, Talajic M. Depression following myocardial infarction: Impact on 6 month survival. J Am Med Assoc 1993; 270:1819–1825.
56. McKelvie RS, Teo KK, McCartney N, Humen D, Montague T, Yusuf S. Effects of exercise training in patients with congestive heart failure: a critical review. J Am Coll Cardiol 1995; 25:789–796.
57. Coats AJS, Adamopoulos S, Radaelli A, McConce A, Meyer TE, Bernardi L, Solda PL, Davey P, Omerod O, Forfar C, Conway J, Sleight P. Controlled trial of physical training in chronic heart failure: exercise performance, hemodynamic ventilation and autonomic function. Circulation 1992; 85:2119–2131.
58. Bittner V, Weiner DH, Yusuf S, Rogers WJ, McIntyre KM, Bangdiwala SI, Kronenberg MW, Kostis JB, Kohn RM, Guillotte M, Greenberg B, Woods PA, Bourassa MG. Prediction of mortality and morbidity with a six-minute walk test in patients with left ventricular dysfunction. J Am Med Assoc 1993; 270:1702–1707.

10

Estrogen Replacement Therapy and Cardiovascular Disease

Laura P. Fowlkes and Jay M. Sullivan

University of Tennessee, Memphis
Memphis, Tennessee

Although there has been an encouraging decrease in the death rate from coronary heart disease over the past quarter century, the incidence is sill very high, causing over 500,000 deaths per year in the United States alone. Much attention is given to known risk factors such as cigarette smoking, hypertension, and hypercholesterolemia, but only recently has the impact of the menopause been widely appreciated.

Data from the Framingham cohort clearly indicate that there are sex-specific differences in the manifestations of coronary heart disease (1). Women have a delay in onset of coronary disease by 10 years relative to men. Myocardial infarction and sudden death are delayed by 20 years. Women lose their resistance to coronary disease as the menopause progresses. The Framingham cohort exhibited a greater than twofold age-adjusted increase in risk for coronary heart disease in postmenopausal women compared to premenopausal women (2).

The effect of hormone replacement therapy in coronary heart disease in postmenopausal women remains a subject of intense debate. Many studies have been performed utilizing various designs and yielding at times conflicting conclusions. This chapter attempts to discuss the consensus to date.

Some of the earliest analyses have been hospital-based case–control studies. These studies have consistently failed to show a protective effect. Comorbidity in the control groups made this study design less than ideal. Rosenberg et al. (3) demonstrated that there was no significant protective effect in 477 women aged 30–49 who were hospitalized for myocardial infarction compared to 1832 hospitalized controls. The control group included a significant number of patients with fractures. The large number of fractures in the controls may have been a marker of decreased exposure to estrogens, raising the question of an exposure bias that would underestimate the protective effect of estrogens.

Jick and colleagues (4) reported an adverse effect in 17 women under age 46 who were admitted for myocardial infarction compared to 34 hospitalized controls. Of the cases, only one had never smoked. The small study size and the possible confounding effect of smoking made it difficult to determine whether the adverse cardiovascular effect noted by the investigators was indeed related to estrogen use.

Community-based studies avoided many of the potential sources of bias in the hospital-based studies. These studies routinely matched patients admitted to the hospital for myocardial infarction or who died form a coronary event to controls from the same community. Using pharmacy records to document estrogen exposure, Pfeffer and associates (5) reported a nonsignificant protective effect in 15,500 women aged 57–98 who lived in a retirement community in California.

Ross and associates (6) subsequently studied the same community. They noted a greater accuracy in determining estrogen exposure when the criteria were based on medical records rather than pharmacy records. The relative risk estimate of death from ischemic heart disease in estrogen users compared to living controls was 0.43 (CI 0.24–0.75; $p < 0.01$); compared to deceased controls it was 0.57 (CI 0.33–0.99; $p < 0.05$). With the exception of the study by Ross et al., none of the community-based studies was able to show a statistically significant benefit. There was, however, a suggestion of a protective effect.

Some investigators have used angiography to study the prevalence of significant coronary artery disease in women based on estrogen use. Gruchow and his coworkers (7) analyzed data obtained from 933 postmenopausal women in the Milwaukee Cardiovascular Data Registry who underwent coronary angiography. The odds ratio for estrogen use was calculated for patients for low, moderate, and severe angiographic occlusion scores and was adjusted for age, smoking, exercise, and body mass. Women with low occlusion scores served as the referent group. Those with moderate occlusion scores had an odds ratio for estrogen use of 0.59 (CI 0.48–0.73), and those with severe occlusion scores an odds ratio of 0.37 (CI 0.29–0.46). Thus, women with severe disease were least likely to use estrogen. Three additional angiographic studies have found that there is a decreased prevalence of angiographic coronary artery disease in estrogen users (8–10).

To analyze the role of blood lipids, Gruchow and colleagues (7) employed a statistical model treating lipids as possible explanatory variables. The estrogen users had significantly higher HDL cholesterol values than did the nonusers. The inclusion of HDL cholesterol in this model reduced the negative association between estrogen use and occlusion score so that the relationship was no longer statistically significant, suggesting that the effect of estrogen on coronary artery disease was partially mediated by HDL cholesterol.

Several important prospective studies have yielded statistically significant protective effects. Bush and colleagues (11) demonstrated a 66% reduction in the incidence of death from major coronary events in 2270 females aged 40–69 evaluated over

8.5 years. Estrogen users had higher mean HDL and lower LDL cholesterol levels compared to nonusers. When HDL cholesterol was added to the regression model, the protective effect of estrogen was attenuated by greater than 40%, suggesting that HDL cholesterol was partially responsible for the protective effect.

Stampfer and coworkers (12) reported results form the Nurses' Health Study. Compared with never-users of postmenopausal hormones, the age-adjusted relative risk of CAD in ever-users was 0.5 (CI 0.3–0.8; $p = 0.007$). The risk estimate in current users was 0.3 (CI 0.2–0.6; $p = 0.001$). Risk estimates were similar when adjusted for risk factors. The protective effect of estrogens was confirmed in the 10-year follow-up from The Nurses' Health Study (13). Henderson and associates (14) demonstrated a protective effect in a population with a mean age of 73 in a large retirement community in California.

One cohort study showed an adverse effect with the use of estrogens in cardiovascular disease. Wilson and associates (15) studied the effect of estrogen use in the Framingham cohort of postmenopausal females aged 50–83 years who participated in the 12th biennial exams and were followed for 8 years. Endpoints were grouped in certain analyses. For example, coronary heart disease included angina pectoris, myocardial infarction, and coronary death or sudden death. Wilson and coworkers reported an age- and risk-factor-adjusted relative-risk estimate for total cardiovascular disease of 1.76 ($p < 0.01$) and for myocardial infarction of 1.87, which was not statistically significant. When patients were grouped according to smoking status, the increased risk for myocardial infarction was statistically significant only in the subgroup who smoked.

Interpretation of the results of the study is limited by several factors. It is known that angina pectoris is not a specific indicator of coronary artery disease, and therefore most studies of estrogen replacement therapy limit the endpoints to events such as fatal and nonfatal myocardial infarction. The investigators also controlled for HDL cholesterol among the other coronary heart disease risk factors. As other studies have shown, adding HDL to the risk-factor-adjusted risk estimate will attenuate and thus underestimate the protective effect of estrogens.

A reanalysis of the Framingham Heart Study (16) eliminated angina pectoris as an endpoint, and noted that the relationship between estrogen replacement therapy and cardiovascular disease noted by Wilson and colleagues (15) was applicable only to the 12th biennial exam. Eaker and Castelli (16) analyzed the data from exams 11 and 12. They demonstrated that in women aged 50–59, there was a protective effect that did not achieve statistical significance. In women aged 60–69 there was an adverse effect that did not achieve statistical significance. The second analysis also controlled for HDL cholesterol, which may result in an underestimate of the protective effect of estrogens.

Until now, there has been only one small randomized trial, by Nachtigall and associates (17), which compared 84 matched pairs of women who were hospitalized in a long-term care facility in New York. There was a nonsignificant reduction in the incidence of myocardial infarction in the estrogen-treated group. The increased incidence of chronic disease and immobility makes the results of the study difficult to extrapolate to the general population.

The effect of estrogen replacement therapy on survival in 2268 women who had undergone angiography and were at risk for coronary artery disease was studied by Sullivan and co-workers (18). Subjects were divided into those who had no, mild to moderate, or severe disease. Five-year survival for the patients without coronary disease was 98% in both users and nonusers. Ten-year survival was 91% in the never-users and 98% in the users (Figure 1). The difference was not statistically significant. Among patients with mild to moderate coronary lesions at baseline, 5-year survival in the never-users was 91% and 10-year survival was 85%. In the ever-users, 5-year survival was 98% and the 10-year survival 96% ($p = 0.027$) (Figure 2). The difference in survival was most marked in those patients with severe lesions. Five-year survival was 81% in the never-users and 60% at 10 years, while 5- and 10-year survival in the ever-users was 98%

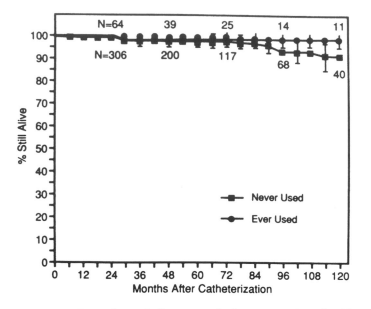

Figure 1   Data from Sullivan et al. demonstrating the 10-year cumulative survival of control patients in the Baptist Memorial Hospital Registry with normal coronary angiograms. Actuarial methods were used to calculate survival. The number of persons still being followed up is indicated by numbers on the survival curves. (From Ref. 18. Arch Intern Med 1990; 150:2557–2562. Copyright 1990, American Medical Association.)

($p = 0.007$) (Figure 3). However, the number of patients in this group of estrogen users was relatively small. The only significant factor predicting survival was estrogen use. Relative risk equaled 0.16 (CI 0.04–0.66).

Stampfer and Colditz (19) reviewed the evidence from 31 studies that had been published and noted that 25 of them showed a protective effect, which was statistically significant in 12. The cumulative relative risk, including all studies based on ever-use of estrogen, was 0.56 (0.50–0.61).

The most accurate reflections of the true effect were felt to be in the two study designs using angiography and the prospective

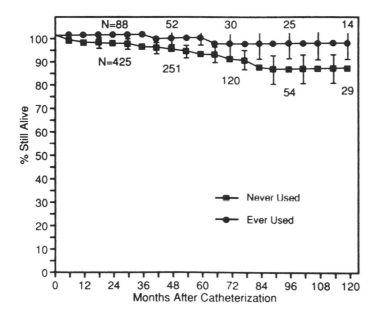

Figure 2 Data from Sullivan et al. demonstrating the 10-year survival of group 1 patients from the Baptist Memorial Hospital Registry whose coronary stenosis varied between detectable and 69%. (From Ref. 18. Arch Intern Med 1990; 150:2557–2562. Copyright 1990, American Medical Association.)

studies with internal control groups. The combined relative-risk estimate for the two study designs was 0.50 (CI 0.43–0.56) (Figure 4).

In their discussion, Stampfer and Colditz (19) commented that, while the prospective studies with internal control groups and the angiography studies appear to come closest to measuring the degree of protection offered by estrogens, these studies are not without potential sources of bias. The question can be raised whether users of estrogens are healthier at baseline and that is why they suffer fewer cardiac events. However, several of the better-designed prospective studies chose control groups that were similar in risk-factor profiles to the cases (11,12,14,15), and

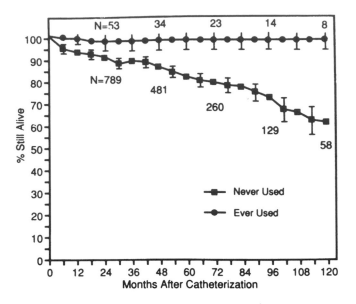

Figure 3 Data from Sullivan et al. demonstrating the 10-year survival of group 2 patients from the Baptist Memorial Hospital Registry with left main coronary stenosis of 50% or greater, or other stenosis of 70% or greater. (From Ref. 18. Arch Intern Med 1990; 150:2557–2562. Copyright 1990, American Medical Association.)

multivariate analysis failed to significantly change the risk estimate.

Several authors have attempted to control for frequency of clinic visits to address the issue of whether estrogen users simply are more vigilant about their health care, and this is the reason they have fewer cardiac events (6,13). As noted by Stampfer and Colditz (19), greater contact with health care providers would tend to document more coronary events in the user groups, which would result in an underestimate of the protective effect. Thus, it would seem unlikely that a protective effect was noted simply because estrogen users were healthier or more vigilant about their health care.

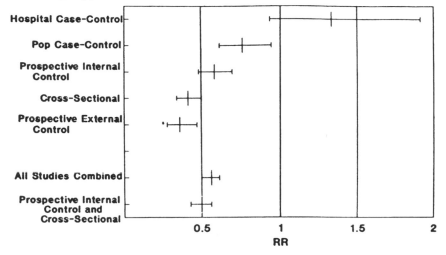

Figure 4 Data presented by Stampfer and Colditz demonstrating summary relative risks and 95% confidence interval estimates for studies of estrogen use and risk of coronary disease, by study design. There was significant ($p < 0.001$) heterogeneity by study design. (From Ref. 19.)

Stampfer and Colditz (19) note that the pooled data failed to demonstrate a convincing trend in estrogen's protective effect based on duration of use, and that there was no clear dose-response effect. Current users experienced more protection than past users. Current and past use was superior to never-use. With rare exceptions (20), most studies reveal that the protective effect of estrogens is conveyed to women with both natural and surgical menopause (7,13,14).

Previous evidence suggests that an important part of the cardioprotective effect of estrogen replacement therapy is due to an effect on serum lipids. It is known that many postmenopausal women have an HDL cholesterol level less than 46 mg/dl, which is associated with a sixfold higher risk of coronary disease than that in women who have HDL cholesterol values greater than 67 mg/dl (21). LDL cholesterol rises with age and is higher in older women than in men. Data from Bush and Miller (22) demonstrated that conjugated estrogens in menopausal replacement doses (0.625 mg) increased total cholesterol by 1%, increased HDL cholesterol by 10%, increased triglycerides by 11%, and decreased LDL cholesterol by 4%. It is postulated that those women who require either cyclic or daily supplementation with progestins would experience an attenuation of the beneficial effect. Sherwin and Gelfand (23) reported that the daily administration of conjugated equine estrogens (CEE) with the cyclic coadministration of medroxyprogesterone acetate (MPA) attenuated but did not completely reverse the beneficial lipid effects of estrogens. Other investigators have confirmed the acceptability of this approach (24,25).

The interaction of estrogens on lipoprotein pathways is complex. Estrogen increases the activity of hepatic apoprotein B and E receptors, increases the uptake of LDL cholesterol and chylomicron remnants, and thus decreases LDL levels. By increasing the synthesis of apoprotein A1 and reducing the activity of hepatic lipoprotein lipase, estrogen raises HDL cholesterol levels (26).

Additional effects on lipoproteins are being evaluated in an effort to explain the relationship of estrogens, menopause, and protection from ischemic heart disease. One of those is lipoprotein (a), which is a complex between LDL and apolipoprotein (a) and is known to be an independent predictor of premature coronary disease (27). There is evidence from investigators in Milan, Italy (28), suggesting that treatment with menopausal replacement doses of CEE may improve lipid profiles by decreasing Lp(a) concentration.

Estrogen replacement therapy increases the risk of endometrial cancer, a risk that is greatly reduced by the addition of progestin. However, progestins attenuate the HDL cholesterol–elevating properties of estrogens, according to a number of short-term studies. In nonhuman primates, both estrogen and estrogen with progestin were found to reduce the extent of aortic atherosclerosis in surgically menopausal monkeys fed a high-fat diet, even though HDL levels were reduced by combination therapy (29).Combination therapy also reduced LDL cholesterol uptake by blood-vessel cells to the same extent as estrogen replacement therapy.

In long-term human cohort studies, such as the Rancho Bernardo Study (30) and the Atherosclerosic Risk in Communities Study (31), HDL levels did not differ significantly between those receiving estrogen and those receiving combined hormone replacement therapy. A recent Swedish cohort study (32) showed approximately equal reduction of cardiovascular risk in women receiving estrogen and those receiving combination replacement. The single published randomized trial of estrogen replacement, that of Nachtigall et al. (17), showed a reduction in the rate of myocardial infarction in hospitalized women who received combination therapy. However, the results of two current, larger, prospective placebo-controlled trials of hormone replacement therapy for cardiovascular endpoints will not be available for years.

In recent years it has been learned that the endothelium plays an important role in the modulation of blood-vessel tone. Furchgott and Zawadzk (33) were the first to demonstrate that the response of normal healthy vessels to acetylcholine stimulation was vasodilation while, after removal of the endothelium, acetylcholine caused vasoconstriction. Subsequently it has been discovered that acetylcholine occupies receptors on the endothelial cell membrane that stimulate the release of endothelial-derived relaxing factor, a vasodilatory, platelet-repelling compound. Relaxing factor is now known to be, either wholly or partially, nitric oxide (34).

Ludmer and colleagues (35) demonstrated that acetylcholine, infused into normal human coronary arteries, caused vasodilation whereas infusion of the same dose in a segment of the artery with an atherosclerotic lesion resulted in vasoconstriction of the diseased and adjacent areas. More recently, Williams and colleagues (36) have demonstrated that when oophorectomized monkeys are fed a high-lipid diet, acetylcholine causes coronary vasoconstriction when infused into the coronary vessels. However, when these monkeys received estrogen replacement therapy, the infusion of acetylcholine caused vasodilation as it does in normal animals. Similar observations have been reported in women (37). Thus, there is evidence that estrogens influence endothelial cell function, and this may play a part in their cardioprotective effect.

Thus far, during this discussion, only the cardiovascular benefits of estrogen replacement therapy have been considered. While there are other benefits, there are risks as well. Grady and colleagues (38) reported results from a meta-analysis assessing the risks and benefits of use of hormone replacement therapy in preventing disease and prolonging life in asymptomatic white postmenopausal women 50 years old. Pooled relative-risk estimates from published studies of ever-use of estrogen compared to never-use yielded relative-risk estimates of 2.31 (CI 2.13–2.51) for endometrial carcinoma, 1.01 (CI 0.97–1.05) for breast cancer, 0.65 (CI 0.59–0.71) for coronary heart disease, 0.75 (0.68–0.84) for hip fracture, and 0.96 (0.82–1.13) for stroke. The only disease for which there were enough data to yield a pooled relative-risk estimate for combined estrogen and progestin use was endometrial carcinoma, for which there was no increased risk with combination therapy.

Changes in overall life expectancy were calculated. In women without a uterus, the life expectancy for unopposed estrogen increased by 1.1 years. In women with an intact uterus, life expectancy increased by 0.9 years. To calculate the effects of adding a progestin to life expectancy, two scenarios were compared. If progestins were postulated to have no effect on overall mortality, life expectancy increased by a full 1.0 year. When a more pessimistic effect was tested—by assigning the relative risk of dying from ischemic heart disease of 0.80 instead of the predicted 0.65 with unopposed estrogens, and by using a relative-risk estimate for breast cancer of 2.0 as opposed to 1.01—the increase in life expectancy was reduced to 0.10 years. Grady and coworkers (38) concluded that estrogen replacement therapy was beneficial to women without intact uteri who were at risk for or had coronary disease, and that there was insufficient evidence that women without coronary disease and those with intact uteri would obtain substantial survival benefits from hormone replacement therapy.

Studies are underway that will address these issues. However, in the case of primary prevention, answers will not be obtained for many years. For the present, the use of estrogen replacement therapy is a decision that must be made between the patient and her physician on an individual basis, weighing the risks and benefits.

REFERENCES

1. Lerner DJ, Kannel WB. Patterns of coronary heart disease morbidity and mortality in the sexes: A 26-year follow-up of the Framingham population. Am Heart J 1986; 383–390.
2. Kannel WB. Metabolic risk factors for coronary heart disease in women: Perspective from the Framingham Study. Am Heart J 1987; 114:413–419.
3. Rosenberg L, Slone D, Shapiro S, et al. Noncontraceptive estrogens and myocardial infarction in young women. JAMA 1980; 244: 339–342.
4. Jick H, Dinan B, Rothman KJ. Noncontraceptive estrogens and nonfatal myocardial infarction. JAMA 1978; 239:1407–1408.
5. Pfeffer RI, Whipple GH, Kurosaki TT, et al. Coronary risk and estrogen use in postmenopausal women. Am J Epidemiol 1978; 107:479–487.
6. Ross, RK, Paganini-Hill A, Mack TM, et al. Menopausal oestrogen therapy and protection from death from ischemic heart disease. Lancet 1981; i:858–860.
7. Gruchow HW, Anderson AJ, Barboriak JJ, et al. Postmenopausal use of estrogen and occlusion of coronary arteries. Am Heart J 1988; 115:954–963.
8. Sullivan JM, Vander Zwaag R, Lemp GF, et al. Postmenopausal estrogen use and coronary atherosclerosis. Ann Intern Med 1988; 108:358–363.
9. McFarland KF, Boniface ME, Hornung CA, et al. Risk factors and noncontraceptive estrogen use in women with and without coronary disease. Am Heart J 1989; 117:1209–1214.

10. Hong MK, Romm PA, Reagan K, et al. Effects of estrogen replacement therapy on serum lipid values and angiographically defined coronary artery disease in postmenopausal women. Am J Cardiol 1992; 69:176–178.

11. Bush TL, Barrett-Conner E, Cowan LD, et al. Cardiovascular mortality and noncontraceptive use of estrogen in women: Results from the Lipid Research Clinics Program Follow-up Study. Circulation 1987; 75:1102–1109.

12. Stampfer MJ, Willett WC, Colditz GA, et al. A prospective study of postmenopausal estrogen therapy and coronary heart disease. N Engl J Med 1985; 313:1044–1049.

13. Stampfer MJ, Colditz GA, Willitt WC, et al. Postmenopausal estrogen therapy and cardiovascular disease: Ten year follow-up from the Nurses' Health Study. N Engl J Med 1991; 325:756–62.

14. Henderson BE, Paganini-Hill A, Ross RK. Estrogen replacement therapy and protection from acute myocardial infarction. Am J Obstet Gynecol 1988; 159:312–317.

15. Wilson PW, Garrison RJ, Castelli WP. Postmenopausal estrogen use, cigarette smoking, and cardiovascular morbidity in women over 50: The Framingham Study. N Engl J Med 1985; 313:1038–1043.

16. Eaker ED, Castelli WP. Coronary heart disease and its risk factors among women in the Framingham Study. In: Eaker E, Packard B, Wenger NK, Clarkson TB, Tyroler HA, eds. Coronary Heart Disease in Women. New York: Haymarket Doyma 1987:122–132.

17. Nachtigall LE, Nachtigall RH, Nachtigall RD, et al. Estrogen replacement therapy. II: A prospective study in the relationship to carcinoma and cardiovascular and metabolic problems. Obstet Gynecol 1979; 54:74–79.

18. Sullivan JM, Vander Zwaag R, Hughes JP, et al. Estrogen replacement and coronary artery disease-effect on survival in postmenopausal women. Arch Intern Med 1990; 150:2557–2562.

19. Stampfer MJ, Colditz GA. Estrogen replacement therapy and coronary heart disease: a quantitative assessment of the epidemiologic evidence. Prev Med 1991; 20:47–63.

20. Bain C, Willett WC, Henenekens CH, et al. Use of postmenopausal hormones and risk of myocardial infarction. Circulation 1981; 64:42–46.

21. Abbott RD, Wilson PWF, Kannel WB, et al. High density lipopro-

tein cholesterol, total cholesterol screening, and myocardial infarction: The Framingham Study. Arteriosclerosis 1988; 8:207.

22. Bush TL, Miller VT. Effects of pharmacologic agents used during menopause. Impact on lipids and lipoproteins. In: Mishell D, ed. Menopause: Physiology and Pharmacology. Chicago: Year Book Medical Publishers, 1986:187–208.

23. Sherwin BB, Gelfand MM. A prospective one-year study of estrogen and progestin in postmenopausal women: effects on clinical symptoms and lipoprotein lipids. Obstet Gynecol 1989; 73:759–766.

24. Weinstein L. Efficacy of a continuous estrogen-progestin regimen in the menopausal patient. Obstet Gynecol 1987; 69:929–932.

25. Luciano AA, Turksoy RN, Carleo J, et al. Clinical and metabolic responses of menopausal women to sequential versus continuous estrogen and progestin replacement therapy. Obstet Gynecol 1988; 71:39–43.

26. Ettinger B. Hormone replacement therapy and coronary heart disease. Obstet Gynecol Clin North Am 1990; 4:741–757.

27. Rhoads GG, Dahlen G, Berg K, et al. Lp(a) lipoprotein as a risk factor for myocardial infarction. JAMA 1986; 256:2540–2544.

28. Soma M, Fumagalli R, Paoletti R, et al. Plasma Lp(a) concentration after oestrogen and progestogen in postmenopausal women (letter). Lancet 1991; 337:612.

29. Adams MR. Kaplan JR, Manuk SB, et al. Inhibition of coronary artery atherosclerosis by 17B estradiol in ovariectomized monkeys: lack of an effect of added progesterone. Arteriosclerosis 1990; 1051–1057.

30. Barrett-Conner E, Wingard DL, Criqui MH. Postmenopausal estrogen use and heart disease risk factors in the 1980's: Rancho Bernardo, California revisited. JAMA 1989; 267:2095–2100.

31. Nabulsi AA, Folsom AR, White A, et al. Association of hormone-replacement therapy with various cardiovascular risk factors in postmenopausal women. N Engl J Med 1993; 328:1069–1075.

32. Falkeborn M, Persson I, Adami H-O, et al. The risk of acute myocardial infarction after oestrogen and oestrogen-progestogen replacement. Br J Obstet Gynaecol 1992; 99:821–828.

33. Furchgott RF, Zawadzk JV. The obligatory role of endothelial cells in the relaxation of arterial smooth muscle by acetylcholine. Nature 1980; 288:373–376.

34. Ignarro LJ, Byrns RE, Buga GM, et al. Endothelium-derived relax-

ing factor (EDRF) released from artery and vein appears to be nitric oxide (NO) or a closely related species. Fed Proc 1987; 46:644.

35. Ludmer PL, Selwyn AP, Shook TL, et al. Paradoxical vasoconstriction induced by acetylcholine in atherosclerotic coronary arteries. N Engl J Med 1986; 315:1046–1051.

36. Williams JK, Adams MR, Klopfenstein HS. Estrogen modulates responses of atherosclerotic coronary arteries. Circulation 1990; 81: 1680–1687.

37. Herrington M, Braden G, Downes TR, et al. Estrogen modulates coronary vasomotor responses in postmenopausal women with early atherosclerosis (abstr). Circulation 1992; 86:I–619.

38. Grady D, Rubin SM, Petitti DB, et al. Hormone therapy to prevent disease and prolong life in postmenopausal women. Ann Intern Med 1992; 117:1016–37.

11
Hyperlipidemia

Marcello Arca

Istituto di Terapia Medica Sistematica
Università di Roma "La Sapienza"
Rome, Italy

I. INTRODUCTION

Coronary heart disease (CHD) is the most important cause of death in both men and women. Although the onset of CHD is earlier in men than in women, as many women as men ultimately die of CHD (1). Alterations of plasma lipids and lipoprotein levels are common risk factors for CHD and they predispose both men and women to CHD and increased cardiovascular mortality (2). However, lipoprotein risk factors have some special characteristics in women. Current evidence suggests that elevated plasma cholesterol (hypercholesterolemia) is a risk factor for CHD in women (3). The major component of plasma cholesterol that enhances the risk for CHD is the cholesterol in low-density lipo-proteins (LDLs). Compared with men, only limited data are available relating LDL cholesterol and CHD risk in women, and reports are controversial regarding the significance of high LDL cholesterol levels for the risk of CHD in women (4,5). Further-more, high-density lipoprotein (HDL) cholesterol appears to be the major lipid risk factor in women, with increased concentra-tions of HDL being negatively associated with subsequent coro-nary disease in prospective studies (6).

The incidence of hyperlipidemia increases in women after menopause. In fact, more postmenopausal women have high levels of LDL cholesterol than men of the same age (7). Also, the role of some lipoprotein risk factors seems to change after meno-pause. For example, triglycerides are considered a significant, independent predictor of CHD risk in postmenopausal women (6), whereas its significance as a risk factor for premenopausal women as well as for men is greatly debated (8). In addition, it has recently been suggested that women may have more LDL particles, which are less dense and less atherogenic, than men do, but this favorable condition seems to be reverted after meno-pause (9).

Despite the potential importance of hyperlipidemia in post-menopausal women, the mechanisms causing it have received little attention. In this chapter, some of the unique aspects of hyperlipidemia in postmenopausal women are reviewed, and the current guidelines for identification and treatment of hyper-lipidemia in women are discussed.

II. LIPOPROTEIN RISK FACTORS IN WOMEN

In general, coronary risk rises with increases in LDL cholesterol and falls with increases in HDL levels; this holds true in women as well as in men. There are, however, some quantitative differ-ences. Both the Framingham Study (3) and the Donolo-Tel Aviv Study (4) have shown that the risk of coronary disease in women with a total cholesterol concentration below 264 mg/dl did not vary significantly. Conversely, women with a total cholesterol concentration exceeding 265 mg/dl had a rate of coronary events more than three times higher than that of women with the lowest concentration of cholesterol. These results differ markedly from those in men, for several possible reasons. Because women have higher HDL cholesterol levels than men do, more of the total cholesterol is made up of a protective, nonatherogenic cholesterol. In addition, it has been reported that LDL carries more cholesterol molecules per particle as reflected by the presence of a higher cholesterol-to-protein ratio (10). Therefore, it takes more LDL cholesterol, and thus a higher total cholesterol, to reflect a more atherogenic profile. These findings have also been used to explain why LDL cholesterol has been found to be a less powerful predictor of CHD risk in women than in men (11). However, other factors may be involved: Studies in female primates have demonstrated that the presence of circulating estrogen interferes with LDL uptake in the arterial wall (12), and this, in turn, may be related to the antioxidant properties of estrogens (13). Taken together, these findings suggest that, for any given level, LDL is less atherogenic in women than in men.

The Framingham Study (3), the LRC Follow-Up Study (5), and the Donolo-Tel Aviv Study (4) have prospectively evaluated the association of HDL cholesterol with subsequent coronary disease in women. In each of these studies, HDL was found to be a strong, negative, independent predictor of coronary disease. Except for age, low HDL cholesterol in women was the most powerful predictor of cardiovascular death in the LRC Follow-Up Study. Overall, the results of these epidemiological studies indicate that an increment of 10 mg/dl in HDL cholesterol is associated with a 30–50% reduction of cardiovascular risk in women.

In premenopausal women and in men of all age groups, triglyceride levels do not appear to be a statistically independent predictor of coronary risk when HDL and LDL cholesterol are considered in a multivariate analysis (8). In contrast, triglycerides appear to be an independent predictor of coronary risk in postmenopausal women (5).

III. EFFECT OF MENOPAUSE ON
LIPOPROTEIN RISK FACTORS

Menopause, either natural or surgical, appears to increase the risk of cardiovascular disease in women (14). It has been suggested that the adverse changes in lipids and lipoproteins occurring after menopause may be partly responsible for this increased risk. Several studies have evaluated the association of menopause with changes in lipid and lipoprotein concentrations, by either comparing postmenopausal women with premenopausal controls or comparing menstruating and menopausal women of the same chronological ages. An extensive review (15) of the results of these studies clearly indicates that postmenopausal women tend to have a more atherogenic lipoprotein profile, showing higher plasma levels of cholesterol, triglycerides, LDLs, and very-low-density lipoproteins (VLDLs). These observations have been confirmed in longitudinal follow-ups (16).

One of the most striking phenomena is the change in the concentration of total and LDL cholesterol after menopause. It has been well demonstrated in epidemiological studies that, until about age 55, LDL cholesterol levels are lower in women than in men. After age 55, the relationship is reversed; from then on, women have higher LDL levels than do men of the same age (17).

Because HDL appears to be the most important lipid risk factor for women, the effects of menopause on HDL plasma levels are very important. Unfortunately, few data are available. A prospective study (16) showed that serum levels of HDL cholesterol declined by 6% in women after menopause who did not receive hormone replacement therapy. This decline in HDL was accompanied by a rise in apolipoprotein AI levels, implying a change in the HDL composition (16).

Menopause seems to have a smaller effect on the concentration of plasma triglycerides. Matthews et al. (16) reported a statistically significant increase of total plasma triglyceride levels by 8% in women who became menopausal. However, this increase was only slightly larger than that observed in premenopausal controls (+6%), and the difference disappeared after controlling for age and body mass index. Nonetheless, it would be erroneous to conclude from these results that hypertriglyceridemia is unimportant as a risk factor in postmenopausal women. As mentioned before, triglyceride levels appear to be independently associated with CHD risk in postmenopausal, but not premenopausal, women (5). However, this may not be a direct consequence of triglycerides. High triglyceride levels are associated with the appearance of a small, dense, more easily oxidized form of LDL (18). It has been reported that this form of LDL is more prominent in older women (9).

Cross-sectional studies have demonstrated that Lp(a) increases after menopause, suggesting that this factor may play a role in the CHD risk at this age (19). However, no direct proof of such a role is available at the moment.

As consequence of these adverse changes, the incidence of all forms of hyperlipidemia increases after menopause. In fact, it has been estimated that in the United States more than 40% of women over age 50 are hypercholesterolemic (7). In view of the importance of hypercholesterolemia in postmenopausal women, it is particularly important to determine the factors underlying this lipid disorder.

IV. FACTORS CAUSING HYPERCHOLESTEROLEMIA IN POSTMENOPAUSAL WOMEN

A. Genetic Factors

Several studies indicate that genetic factors may cause elevation of plasma concentrations of LDL cholesterol. A classic example is familial hypercholesterolemia (FH), in which mutations in the gene coding for the LDL receptor cause an accumulation of LDL due to a reduced catabolism of these lipoproteins. However, there is no evidence for a sex-related inheritance of this genetic form of hypercholesterolemia (20).

The gene coding for apolipoprotein E has been demonstrated to significantly affect LDL cholesterol concentration. This apolipoprotein may be present in three isoforms (E2, E3, and E4), E2 being associated with the lowest and E4 with the highest LDL cholesterol levels (21). However, this relationship has been reported in both men and women, and no study described a different distribution of these isoforms between sexes.

A more interesting question is whether there are genetic factors predisposing women to develop hyperlipidemia after menopause. One might speculate, for example, that "mild" mutations in the LDL receptor may became clinically evident in women only after cessation of estrogen production, or that only women carrying apo E4 may experience the largest increase in cholesterol concentration at older ages. However, no data proving any of these hypotheses are available at the moment.

B. Metabolic Factors

In general, the plasma concentration of a lipoprotein is determined by the balance between its rates of synthesis and catabolism. Low-density lipoproteins arise through the metabolism of triglyceride-rich lipoproteins (22). The liver secretes VLDLs, which are converted, in the peripheral circulation, to VLDL remnants after partial hydrolysis of their triglycerides by the action of lipoprotein lipase. Subsequently, VLDL remnants can be taken up by the liver or converted to LDL. LDL particles leave the circulation mainly through a high-affinity process involving specific cellular receptors, the LDL receptors, and this occurs for the most part in the liver (23).

By reinjecting autologous, radiodinated LDLs, it is possible to estimate the kinetics of LDL in vivo. Therefore, as a step toward the understanding of metabolic defects underlying postmenopausal hypercholesterolemia, we have compared the turnover rates of autologous I^{125} LDL in a group of postmenopausal women with mild to severe hypercholesterolemia (LDL cholesterol above 160 mg/dl) with those in a group of normocholesterolemic women, matched for age and sex-hormone status (24).

As expected, in postmenopausal women plasma levels of LDL cholesterol were significantly influenced by metabolic parameters of LDL particles, as demonstrated by the significant correlations between LDL cholesterol levels with both fractional catabolic rates (FCRs) ($r = -0.59$; $p < 0.001$) and synthetic rate of LDL apo B ($r = 0.52$; $p < 0.001$).

However, the major difference in lipoprotein kinetics observed between the two groups of women was a lower FCR of LDL apoB in those with hypercholesterolemia (Table 1). The FCR of LDL apo B, i.e., the fraction of the LDL apo B pool being removed each day, was reduced by 0.351 ± 0.01 pool/day in control women to 0.290 ± 0.01 pool/day in those with hypercholesterolemia, and this difference was highly statistically significant ($p < 0.001$). All but two control women showed FCR values above 0.30 pools/day, whereas all but five hypercholesterolemic women exhibited FCRs equal or below 0.30 pools/day (Figure 1). No differences were observed in the synthetic rate of LDL apo B (Table 1), and the distribution of individual values was almost identical between the two groups of women (Figure 1).

Table 1 Plasma Concentrations and Kinetic Rates of LDL apo B in Postmenopausal Women with Hypercholesterolemia Compared with Those with Normocholesterolemia

	Postmenopausal Women	
	With hyper-cholesterolemia ($n = 24$)	With normo-cholesterolemia ($n = 13$)
LDL cholesterol (mg/dl)	185.0 ± 23.0[a]	128.0 ± 15.0
LDL apo B (mg/dl)	113.4 ± 3.1[a]	81.0 ± 3.3
Pool size (mg)	2947.4 ± 98.0[a]	2016.5 ± 105.8
Fractional catabolic rate (pools/day)	0.29 ± 0.01[a]	0.35 ± 0.01
Input rate (mg/kg/day)	12.3 ± 0.6	11.1 ± 0.6
Input rate (mg/kg IBW/day)	15.7 ± 0.7	13.6 ± 0.8

Data are reported as M ± SE. IBW (ideal body weight) calculated according to Metropolitan Life Insurance Company tables.
[a]$p < 0.001$ for the comparison with women with normocholesterolemia.
Source: Modified from Ref. 24.

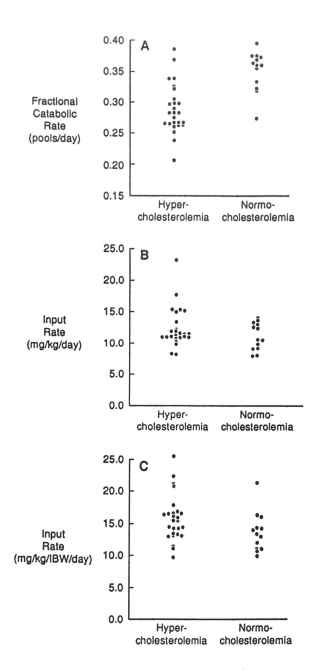

Thus, in our study, hypercholesterolemia in postmenopausal women appeared to be attributable mainly to a reduced catabolism of LDL.

It has been hypothesized that changes in the composition of LDL particles may affect its affinity for the LDL receptor (25). Moreover, it has recently been reported that alterations in the structure of apo B can cause hypercholesterolemia by making LDL particles unable to bind to the receptor (26). Thus, the reduced FCR of LDL observed in our hypercholesterolemic women might have been due to altered receptor-binding properties of their LDL. When this hypothesis was tested directly in transgenic mice for the human LDL receptor, we did not observe any reduction in the binding affinity of LDL isolated from hypercholesterolemic women (unpublished data). In addition, no correlations were observed between the kinetic parameters of LDL apoB and the cholesterol/protein ratio of LDL. Therefore, the most plausible explanation for the reduced clearance of LDL in hypercholesterolemic women is a reduction of LDL receptor activity.

We have considered the possibility that mutations in the LDL receptor gene could account for such reduced activity. To investigate this point we screened hypercholesterolemic women for mutations in the LDL receptor gene by using a combination of single-stranded conformation polymorphism (SSCP) and direct sequencing. None of them showed a structural defect in the LDL receptor gene, leaving the possibility that they may have a metabolic down-regulation of LDL receptor activity.

Figure 1 Individual values of fractional catabolic rate (FCR) and input rate (IR) for LDL apo B in postmenopausal women with hypercholesterolemia and in those with normocholesterolemia. FCRs are expressed as pools of plasma apo B removed per day (pools/day); IRs are expressed as mg of LDL apo B produced per day per kilograms of actual body weight (mg/kg/day) or per kilograms of ideal body weight (mg/kg IBW/day). Ideal body weights were calculated according to the Metropolitan Life Insurance Company tables.

The question then arises of why some postmenopausal women have a suppression of LDL receptor activity. The answer is a matter of speculation. Weight gain after menopause is a common phenomenon, and may predispose women to develop elevated LDL cholesterol levels (27). Obesity has been reported to be associated with reduced catabolism of LDL (28). However, in our group of women, we did not observe any effect of body weight on either LDL cholesterol concentration or kinetic parameters of LDL apo B. It has been suggested that the apo E phenotype may modulate LDL metabolism (21). However, in our small group of women, we have not been able to detect any significant association of the apo E phenotype with kinetic parameters of LDL. Further investigations to clarify this point are needed.

It has been suggested that a decrease in estrogen secretion with cessation of ovarian function probably contribute to higher LDL cholesterol levels in postmenopausal women, and, in those with genetic propensity, loss of estrogen may have raised LDL levels to the high-risk range. In animals (29) and humans (30), estrogens have been shown to stimulate synthesis of LDL receptors, and in humans estrogen therapy lowers LDL cholesterol levels. However, in our study, the lack of estrogens was similar in both groups of postmenopausal women, and thus other factors seem to be responsible for the down-regulation of LDL receptor activity in hyperlipemic women.

Previous studies have reported that primary moderate hypercholesterolemia in middle-aged men is kinetically heterogeneous; several different patterns of abnormal LDL metabolism were found to account for high LDL levels in men (31). However, this heterogeneity in LDL kinetics was not observed in women. Apparently, a reduction in the activity of LDL receptor is the abnormality primarily responsible for hypercholesterolemia in women.

The findings of our study may have some practical implications. They suggest that a selective intervention aimed at up-regulating LDL receptor activity might be the most rational therapeutic approach to controlling high-risk LDL cholesterol levels in older women.

V. IS TREATMENT OF HYPERLIPIDEMIA IN POSTMENOPAUSAL WOMEN BENEFICIAL?

Growing evidence indicates that treatment of lipoprotein disorders may be beneficial in preventing coronary events, not only in men but also in women. A meta-analysis of three interventional studies carried out in the late 1960s and early 1970s demonstrates that equivalent cholesterol lowering in women was associated with equivalent reductions in coronary death rates (32). In addition, aggressive LDL cholesterol lowering and HDL cholesterol raising in severely hypercholesterolemic men and women have been shown to inhibit progression of CHD and induce regression of coronary disease in both sexes (33). Moreover, the Scandinavian Simvastatin Survival Study recently reported that cholesterol-lowering treatment in hyperlipemic women reduces coronary events by 35% (34).

As the risk of CHD related to high plasma LDL cholesterol concentrations is attenuated in older persons, it is not unreasonable to ask whether cholesterol-lowering therapy has the same importance in preventing CHD in postmenopausal women. On the other hand, the benefits of lowering plasma lipid concentrations could be larger in women in their 60s and 70s, given their age-related increase in the risk of CHD. Moreover, the stabilization of atherosclerotic lesions may be of primary importance in the elderly, in whom advanced lesions are common. Therefore, despite the lack of data from controlled clinical trials, efforts to control hyperlipidemia in postmenopausal women appear to be justified. Further support for this position can be found in observational studies reporting lower rates of CHD in postmenopausal women receiving estrogen replacement therapy (35). It is well known that this treatment is able to reduce the concentrations of atherogenic lipoproteins (36).

VI. CURRENT GUIDELINES FOR THE TREATMENT OF HYPERLIPDEMIA IN POSTMENOPAUSAL WOMEN

The new National Cholesterol Education Program (NECP) (37) reports the guidelines for an appropriate treatment of hyper- lipidemia in women to decrease the CHD risk (Table 2). These guidelines confirm LDL as the primary target of intervention in both men and women. However, the statement about gender as a risk factor for CHD has been revised. It is now recognized that women also suffer from this disease, and that only a decade separates its development in women from that in men. Therefore, hypercholesterolemic men above age 45 and women above age 55 should be considered candidates for intervention. This implies that postmenopausal women are regarded as a high-risk group. As far as drug intervention is concerned, these guidelines set an LDL threshold for postmenopausal women of 190 mg/dl, which is higher than the upper limit for men. In this way, the guidelines attempt to account for the fact that the risk of CHD is lower in women than in men throughout most of their lifespan, and that drug intervention should be more limited in women than in men.

Table 2 Classification and Management of Hypercholesterolemia in Women According to the Categories of the National Cholesterol Education Program (NECP)

Categories	Total cholesterol (mg/dl)	LDL cholesterol (mg/dl)
Very high	>265	>190
High	>240	>160
Desirable	<200	<130

Drug therapy guidelines: those with LDL cholesterol >190 mg/dl after diet and those with LDL cholesterol >160 mg/dl after diet in the presence of CHD or two other risk factors.

Source: Adapted from Ref. 37.

The other risk factors that call for full lipoprotein evaluation are the same in men and women—cigarette smoking, hypertension, diabetes, or a family history of CHD. The protective role of HDL has been acknowledged, and low HDL cholesterol concentrations (<35 mg/dl) have been included in the list of additional risk factors for both men and women (Table 3).

There are no differences between men and women with regard to lowering hypertriglyceridemia, and pharmacological treatment is recommended only if other lipoprotein abnormalities are present.

VII. TREATMENT OF HYPERLIPIDEMIA IN POSTMENOPAUSAL WOMEN

A. Dietary Intervention

Dietary therapy is clearly the first step in the management of hyperlipidemia in postmenopausal women, and may lower cholesterol enough to eliminate the need for drug therapy. Although low-cholesterol, low-saturated-fat diets are effective in reducing

Table 3 Evaluation of Risk Status in Women Based on Presence of CHD Risk Factors Other than LDL Cholesterol

Positive risk factors
Age >55 years
Premature menopause without estrogen replacement therapy
Family history of premature CHD
Current cigarette smoking
Hypertension
Low HDL cholesterol (<35 mg/dl)
Diabetes mellitus
Negative risk factors[a]
High HDL cholesterol (>60 mg/dl)

[a]If HDL cholesterol is >60 mg/dl, subtract one risk factor.
Source: Modified from Ref. 37.

LDL cholesterol in women as well as in men, the magnitude of such a decrease appears to be somewhat smaller in women than in men (15). In a large study, almost 2000 normolipidemic, postmenopausal women fed a low-fat, low-cholesterol diet experienced a reduction of LDL of about 20% after 3 weeks of dietary treatment (38). This decline was lower than that obtained in men of comparable ages. However, the cholesterol-lowering potential of such a diet in postmenopausal women with hyperlipidemia remains to be evaluated.

B. Drug Treatment

A recent report of the third National Health and Nutrition Examination Survey indicated that 16 to 23% of postmenopausal women in the United States will be candidates for cholesterol-lowering therapy after a trial of dietary therapy (39). Because a decrease in the activity of LDL receptors appears to be a major cause of hypercholesterolemia in postmenopausal women, a regimen that specifically increases LDL receptor activity may be considered the treatment of choice. Estrogen replacement is one of these. Granfone et al. (40) reported a 27% reduction in LDL cholesterol levels in postmenopausal, hyperlipemic women after 13 weeks of treatment with 0.02 mg/day of ethinyl estradiol. However, these women experienced a significant increase in the concentration of total triglyceride. This treatment has some other limitations and may therefore not be appropriate for all women or may not provide sufficient LDL-lowering for those at high risk. For these reasons, estrogen replacement therapy is considered an intermediate therapy between diet and lipid-lowering drugs.

An alternative approach could be the use of HMG-CoA reductase inhibitors, which have been demonstrated to both up-regulate LDL receptor activity and increase the removal rate of LDL (41). To evaluate the efficacy of such an approach, we carried out a double-blind, controlled study with 16 postmenopausal women with hypercholesterolemia randomized to low-dose (10 mg/d) lovastatin, an HMGCoA reductase inhibitor, or placebo (24). This trial had a crossover design, with each of the two phases lasting 8 weeks. A low dose was chosen for reasons of safety and cost-effectiveness. The effects of lovastatin therapy on plasma lipids and lipoprotein cholesterol levels are shown in Table 4. On average, total cholesterol and LDL cholesterol were reduced by 19% and 22%, respectively, during lovastatin therapy. In addition, VLDL+IDL cholesterol decreased by 33% and triglycerides by 16%. Reductions of total apoB, LDL apo B, and VLDL+IDL apo B concentrations paralleled those observed for cholesterol. Most importantly, all women responded well to treatment; their LDL cholesterol levels were reduced from the high-risk to the low-risk range. These results indicate that postmenopausal hypercholesterolemia may be highly responsive to HMGCoA reductase inhibitors, and that even a low dose of the drug may be sufficient in most women.

Table 4 Changes in Plasma Lipids and Lipoproteins During Treatment with Low-Dose Lovastatin in 16 Postmenopausal Women with Hypercholesterolemia

Lipids (mg/dl)	Placebo	Lovastatin
Total cholesterol	272.0 ± 45.0	221.0 ± 40.0[a]
Total triglycerides	177.0 ± 65.0	148.0 ± 53.0[b]
VLDL+IDL cholesterol	51.0 ± 29.0	34.0 ± 16.0[c]
LDL cholesterol	171.0 ± 31.8	134.0 ± 33.0[a]
HDL cholesterol	51.0 ± 13.2	52.0 ± 12.0
VLDL+IDL apo B	21.0 ± 11.0	14.0 ± 6.0[b]
LDL apo B	110.0 ± 22.0	88.0 ± 23.0[a]
Total apo B	132.0 ± 29.0	102.0 ± 27.0[a]

Data are reported as M ± SE. Apo = apolipoprotein.
[a]$p < 0.001$; [b]$p < 0.05$; [c]$p < 0.01$ for the comparison between placebo and lovastatin period by a two-tailed paired t test.
Source: Modified from Ref. 24.

VIII. CONCLUSIONS

After menopause, women experience a sharp increase of LDL cholesterol, making hypercholesterolemia the most common form of hyperlipidemia in older women. An investigation of the metabolic mechanisms underlying hypercholesterolemia in post-menopausal women revealed that elevated LDL cholesterol levels in these women are consistently attributable to a reduced catabolism of LDL and may be due to a reduced activity of LDL receptors. This appears to be different from the mechanisms observed in men, in whom several different patterns of abnormal LDL metabolism were found to account for high LDL levels. However, further studies are needed for a better understanding of factors predisposing women to develop hypercholesterolemia after menopause. Current guidelines for detection and treatment of lipoprotein abnormalities recognize that postmenopausal women with hyperlipidemia are a subgroup at particularly high risk for CHD and thus deserve special attention.

Management of hyperlipidemia in postmenopausal women is directed primarily at reducing atherogenic lipoproteins. Currently the primary focus is on plasma LDL cholesterol. Drug treatment may be indicated for postmenopausal women with LDL cholesterol levels above 190 mg/dl. Because decreased activity of LDL receptors appears to be a major cause of hypercholesterolemia in postmenopausal women, the use of an agent that specifically increases LDL receptor activity may be considered the treatment of choice. Both estrogen replacement therapy and HMGCoA reductase inhibitors fall into this category. Estrogens may offer health benefits in addition to reducing CHD risk, but HMGCoA reductase inhibitors may be effective even at low doses, thus reducing the cost and increasing the safety of drug therapy. However, clinical-trial evidence of the benefit of cholesterol-lowering in women is scarce.

A question that is still open is how to manage low levels of HDL cholesterol (hypoalphalipoproteinemia) in postmenopausal women. HDL cholesterol is not considered a primary target of intervention in neither men nor women; rather, individuals with low HDL are simply considered to have an additional risk factor. In view of the evidence suggesting that HDL is a strong predictor of CHD risk in women, a better definition of this lipoprotein disorder in postmenopausal women is required.

REFERENCES

1. Thom TJ, Baker ED, Packard B, et al. Cardiovascular disease mortality among United States women. In: Coronary Heart Disease in Women. New York: Haymarket Doyma, 1987: 31–44.
2. Stamler J, Wentworth D, Neaton J. Is the relationship between serum cholesterol risk of death from CHD continuous or graded? JAMA 1986; 256:2823–2828.
3. Castelli WP, Garrison RJ, Wilson PWF, et al. Incidence of coronary heart disease and lipoprotein cholesterol levels: the Framingham Study. JAMA 1986; 256:2835–2838.
4. Brunner D, Weisbort J, Meshulam N, et al. Relation of serum total cholesterol and high density lipoprotein cholesterol percentage to the incidence of definite coronary events: twenty year follow-up of the Donolo-Tel Aviv Prospective Coronary Artery Disease Study. Am J Cardiol 1987; 591:1271–1276.
5. Bush TL, Barrett-Connor E, Cowan LD, et al. Cardiovascular mortality and noncontraceptive use of estrogen in women: results from the Lipid Research Clinic Program Follow-up Study. Circulation 1987; 75:1102–1109.
6. Bass KM, Newshaffer CJ, Klag MJ, Bush TL. Plasma lipoprotein levels as predictors of cardiovascular death in women. Arch Intern Med 1993; 153:2209–2216.
7. Sempos CT, Cleeman JI, Carrol MD, et al. Prevalence of high blood cholesterol among US adults: an update based on guidelines from the second report of the National Cholesterol Education Program Adult Treatment Panel. JAMA 1993; 269:3009–3014.
8. Austin MA. Plasma triglycerides and coronary heart disease. Arterioscl Thromb 1991; 11:2–14.
9. Campos H, McNamara JR, Wilson PWF, et al. Differences in low density lipoprotein subfractions and apolipoproteins in premenopausal and postmenopausal women. J Clin Endocrinol Metab 1988; 67:30–35.
10. Arca M, Vega GL, Grundy SM. Unpublished observation.

11. Eaker ED, Castelli WP. Coronary heart disease and its risk fac-
     tors among women in the Framingham Study. In: Coronary
     Heart Disease in Women. New York: Haymarket Doyma, 1987:
     122–130.
12. Wagner JD, Clarkson TB, St Clair RW, et al. Estrogen replacement
     therapy (ERT) and coronary artery (CA) atherogenesis in sur-
     gically, postmenopausal cynomolgus monkeys (abstr). Circulation
     1989; 80(suppl II), 331.
13. Rifici VA, Khachadurian AK. The inhibition of low-density lipo-
     protein oxidation by 17-beta estradiol. Metabolism 1992; 41:1110–
     1114.
14. Bush TL. The epidemiology of cardiovascular disease in post-
     menopausal women. Ann NY Acad Sci 1990; 592:263–271.
15. Bush TL, Fried LP, Barrett-Connor E. Cholesterol, lipoproteins and
     coronary heart disease in women. Clin Chem 1988; 34:B60–B70.
16. Matthews KA, Meilahn E, Kuller LH, et al. Menopause and risk
     factors for coronary heart disease. N Engl J Med 1989; 321:641–646.
17. The Expert Panel. Report of the National Cholesterol Education
     Program Expert Panel on detection, evaluation, and treatment of
     high blood cholesterol in adults. Arch Intern Med 1988; 148:36–69.
18. de Graaf J, Hak-Lemmers HLM, Hectors MPC, et al. Enhanced
     susceptibility to in vitro oxidation of the dense low-density lipo-
     protein subfraction in healthy subjects. Arterioscler Thromb 1991;
     11:298–306.
19. Utermann G. The mysteries of lipoprotein(a). Science 1989; 246:
     904–910.
20. Goldstein JL, Brown SM. Familial hypercholesterolemia. In: The
     Metabolic Basis of Inherited Diseases. New York: McGraw-Hill,
     1989:1215–1250.
21. Davignon J, Gregg RE, Sing CF. Apolipoprotein E polymorphism
     and atherosclerosis. Arteriosclerosis 1988; 8:1–21.
22. Havel RJ. The formation of LDL: mechanism and regulation. J
     Lipid Res 1984; 25:157–1576.
23. Brown MS, Goldstein L. A receptor-mediated pathway for choles-
     terol homeostasis. Science 1986; 232:34–47.
24. Arca M, Vega GL, Grundy SM. Hypercholesterolemia in post-
     menopausal women. JAMA 1994; 271:453–459.
25. Witztum JL, Young SG, Elam RL, et al. Cholestyramine-induced
     changes in low density lipoprotein composition and metabolism. I.
     Studies in guinea pigs. J Lipid Res 1985; 26:92–102.

26. Innerarity TL, Mahley RW, Weisgraber KH, et al. Familial defective apolipoprotein B-100: a mutation of lipoprotein B that causes hypercholesterolemia. J Lipid Res 1990; 31:1337– 1349.

27. VanItallie TB. The perils of obesity in middle-aged women. N Engl J Med 1990; 322:928–929.

28. Kasaniemy YA, Grundy SM. Increased low density lipoprotein production associated with obesity. Arteriosclerosis 1983; 3: 170–177.

29. Windler EE, Kovanen PT, Chao YS, et al. The estradiol-stimulated lipoprotein receptor of rat liver: A binding site that mediates the uptake of rat lipoprotein containing apoproteins B and E. J Biol Chem 1980; 255:10464–10471.

30. Eriksson M, Berglund L, Rudling M, et al. Effects of estrogens on low density lipoprotein metabolism in males: short-term and long-term studies during hormonal treatment of prostatic carcinoma. J Clin Invest 1989; 84:802–810.

31. Grundy SM. Multifactorial etiology of hypercholesterolemia: Implications for prevention of coronary heart disease. Arterioscler Thromb 1991; 11:1619–1635.

32. Rossouw JF. International trials: Cholesterol and heart disease in older persons and in women (abstr). Bethesda, MD: National Heart, Lung and Blood Institute, National Institutes of Health, 1990.

33. Kane JP, Malloy MJ, Ports TA, et al. Regression of coronary atherosclerosis during treatment of familial hypercholesterolemia with combined drug regimens. JAMA 1990; 264:3007–3012.

34. Scandinavian Simvastatin Study Group. Randomized trial of cholesterol-lowering in 4444 patients with coronary heart disease: The Scandinavian Simvastatin Survival Study (4S). Lancet 1994; 344:1383–1389.

35. Stampfer MJ, Colditz GA. Estrogen replacement and coronary heart disease: a quantitative assessment of the epidemiologic evidence. Prev Med 1991; 20:47–63.

36. Sacks FM, Walsh BW. Sex hormones and lipoprotein metabolism. Curr Opin Lipidol 1994; 5:236–240.

37. Expert Panel on Detection, Evaluation, and Treatment of High Blood Cholesterol in Adults. Summary of the second report of the National Cholesterol Education Program (NCEP) expert panel on detection, evaluation, and treatment of high blood cholesterol in adults (Adult Treatment Panel II). JAMA 1993; 269:3015–3023.

38. Barnard RF. Effects of life-style modification on serum lipids. Arch Intern Med 1991; 151:1389–1394.

39. The National Health and Nutrition Examination Surveys. Declining serum total cholesterol levels among US adults. JAMA 1993; 269:3002–3008.

40. Granfone A, Campos H, McNamara JR, et al. Effects of estrogen replacement on plasma lipoproteins and apolipoproteins in postmenopausal, dyslipidemic women. Metabolism 1992; 41:1193–1198.

41. Grundy SM. HMG-CoA reductase inhibitors for treatment of hypercholesterolemia. N Engl J Med 1988; 319:24–33.

12

Postmenopausal Hypertension Put into Perspective

Karen D. Bradshaw

University of Texas Southwestern Medical Center
Dallas, Texas

Many women view their gynecologist as their primary physician, at least through their menstrual problems, child bearing, infertility or contraception, and sexual issues, and into menopause. With increasing life expectancy, many women will spend more than one-third of their lifespan in the postmenopausal state. As primary health care providers, gynecologists are in a unique position to provide ongoing care, education, and preventive health counseling as women age. Graceful, healthful aging with an emphasis on prevention and early detection should be a primary concern of all.

The average age of menopause is a mean age of 51, with a normal range of 45–51 years of age. The result of the menopausal ovarian failure is a depletion of oocytes, follicular development, and cyclic ovarian estrogen and progesterone production due to cessation of ovulation. The amenorrhea of menopause may be preceded by several years of anovulatory bleeding. The prime symptoms of the menopause are the final menses, hot flashes, vaginal dryness, and discomfort and bladder symptoms due to vaginal atrophy. A women who lives to be 50 has about a 65% chance of developing hypertension, a 46% lifetime probability of developing heart disease, and a 31% probability of dying from heart disease by about age 74.

Postmenopausal women represent the largest category of women who are at risk for hypertension and coronary heart disease (CHD). The risk for CHD is due not only to the rise in lipid risk factors with age in the non-estrogen-treated postmenopausal women, but also to the rise of other risk factors—most notably, obesity, hypertension, and diabetes—that occur with aging. After menopause, the incidence of hypertension, cardiovascular disease, and cardiovascular mortality increases progressively in women relative to men, leading to an eventual equal incidence in both sexes. Most untreated women with hypertension will develop further increases in their arterial pressure with time, leading to an even greater risk of CHD and other disorders associated with hypertension.

The most frequent cause of death among U.S. women is cardiovascular disease, which results in approximately 250,000 deaths per year. This accounts for 42% of deaths in women over the age of 50. Cummings et al. (1) examined the lifetime risk of certain disease processes in postmenopausal women. They concluded: "The lifetime risk of death due to coronary heart disease is about ten times greater than the risk of either hip fractures or breast cancer." While healthy women with no underlying risk factors who undergo a natural menopause do not appear to be at immediate risk of heart disease, obvious questions arise from studying the relationship of menopause and CHD:

1. Does the menopause alter or modify other risk factors—most importantly, hypertension and lipoproteins—to promote cardiovascular disease at a later period?

2. Are cardiovascular diseases in the 60s and 70s related to delayed manifestations of subclinical events in the immediate menopause?

Several cross-sectional and longitudinal studies have demonstrated that blood pressure increases with age (2–7). In general, epidemiological studies have shown that women under age 40 years have lower systolic pressure than men, but after age 60 years it is higher than that of men. Whether ovarian failure contributes to this rapid rise in systolic pressure has been controversial. In contrast, diastolic pressure increases to a lesser degree with age (8), and no clear difference has been observed between the sexes.

Since there are more elderly women than elderly men, and since hypertension is both more common and deadly in the elderly, more women than men will suffer a cardiovascular complication attributable to hypertension. However, women are somehow protected against death from CHD when compared to men with comparable risk profiles (9); this is likely the most important reason for the longer lifespan of women.

Possible explanations for this protection are as follows:

A protective effect of estrogens, perhaps mediated through higher HDL cholesterol levels
Reduction of blood viscosity and body iron stores by regular menses
Less insulin resistance and hyperinsulinemia because of less upper-body fat
A lower rate of cigarette smoking

It is known that blood pressure alters during the normal menstrual cycle, suggesting that female hormones may affect blood pressure (10,11). Since hypertension is less common in women before menopause than in men, it has been suggested that estrogens in premenopausal women might act as a protective factor for hypertension. This view was confirmed by findings that menopausal women using physiological estrogen replacement had lower blood pressure than did controls (12,13). Estrogen has also been shown to have a direct beneficial effect on vessel-wall physiology in several studies (14–19). The extent to which this may be involved in the development of an "estrogen withdrawal hypertension" is unclear. These findings are confirmed by the Postmenopausal Estrogen/Progestin Interventions (PEPI) Trial (20). This is a 3-year, multicenter, randomized, double-blind, placebo-controlled trial of 875 healthy postmenopausal women designed to assess pairwise differences between the effects of placebo, unopposed estrogen, and three estrogen–progestin regimens on selected heart-disease risk factors. Regarding blood pressure, there were no significant differences in systolic blood pressure among the treatment groups. Mean systolic blood-pressure levels decreased slightly during the first year and increased significantly thereafter in all groups by about 5%, including in women assigned to placebo. Diastolic blood pressure did not vary significantly by treatment assignment. Little change was seen in diastolic pressures over the 3-year study (20).

Messerli et al. (21) studied 100 men and 100 women with mild essential hypertension. Women with essential hypertension were characterized by a higher cardiac index, left ventricular ejection time, and pulse pressure; a slightly faster heart rate; and a lower total peripheral resistance than men with the same arterial pressure. The blood volume of female patients was slightly more contracted than that of male patients, as were the total blood volume and the erythrocyte mass. No differences were noted in resting plasma levels of norepinephrine, epinephrine, dopamine, or plasma renin activity. However, the increase in arterial and pulse pressure caused by isometric stress was almost 50% higher in men than in women. Response of other hemodynamic indices was not significantly different between the two groups.

To evaluate the effects of the menopause, Messerli et al. further subdivided patient pairs into two age groups: those older and those younger than 45 years of age. The difference between men and women in cardiac output and total peripheral resistance was more marked in the younger age group, but was not statistically significant in those pairs of patients who were older than 45 years of age.

The authors concluded that premenopausal women are hemodynamically younger than men of the same chronological age. However, this hemodynamic pattern in women seems to last only until menopause; thereafter the pattern in women was not significantly different from that seen in men. Messerli et al. postulate that estrogen may act to decrease total peripheral resistance and may also be associated with a lower rise in arterial pressure associated with mental stress.

Another possible etiology, although certainly not the whole explanation, is that menstruating women have a lower hematocrit value and a slightly lower fluid volume than either non-menstruating women or men. Their normal hematocrit would be in the range of 37 to 39 instead of 42 to 45. Increased blood viscosity causes an increase in resistance to blood flow, and a reduction in flow can lead to coronary occlusion and increased peripheral resistance, which can contribute to hypertension as seen in polycythemic states (22).

Studies designed to prove or disprove a hypothetical causal relation between loss of ovarian function and rise in blood pressure have yielded conflicting results (23,24). However, early studies did little to separate the effect of chronological aging from that of time of ovarian failure. Another important confounding factor that is not always examined is the effect of changes in body weight and body fat. Several studies (25,26) have demonstrated that changes in blood pressure are positively correlated with changes in body mass index. Cross-sectional studies (3,5) show that women tend to gain more weight between ages 40 and 60 than men, which may be attributed, in part, to changes in hormone production (27) as well as a decline in physical activity associated with aging.

van Beresteijn et al. (28) studied 168 healthy normotensive pre-, peri, and postmenopausal women in Ede, the Netherlands, to see the extent to which ovarian failure and aging contributed to blood pressure. The mixed, longitudinally designed study followed women for 7 years and classified women in birth cohorts (groups of women with the same year of birth) and in menopausal cohorts (groups of women with the same year after menopause). Body mass index and entry blood pressure were studied as confounding factors in multiple regression analyses.

In all chronological age groups, systolic as well as diastolic pressures tended to be negatively related to years since menopause. Positive relationships between changes in blood pressure and changes in body mass index were seen. Their conclusion was that blood pressure does not increase in healthy normotensive perimenopausal women whose body weights are relatively stable.

Wu et al. (29) measured arterial blood pressure, serum lipids, and the fat synergic index in 598 Chinese women aged 40 to 54 years. In their study, menopausal or postmenopausal women had higher mean levels of serum cholesterol, triglycerides, and HDL cholesterol, and had a higher prevalence of hypertension, hypercholesterolemia, and hypertriglyceridemia than premenopausal controls. However, they found no differences in mean values of systolic and diastolic pressures among premenopausal, menopausal, and postmenopausal women. In multiple linear regression analysis, the fat synergic index—(weight × waist circumference)/height—had the strongest association and was positively associated with serum cholesterol and triglyceride levels and systolic and diastolic blood pressure and inversely associated with HDL-cholesterol concentration. Interestingly, of the independent variables studied, progesterone was found to be a protective factor for hypertension.

The relationship between menopause and occurrence of arterial hypertension was evaluated by Taylor et al. (23) in a group of 179 surgically castrated women and 21 women with a natural menopause. No difference between the incidence of hypertension in postmenopausal women and that in the general population was found. The authors concluded that loss of ovarian function is neither a primary nor a contributory factor in arterial hypertension.

Environmental factors are also important, as has been shown in an interesting study by Timio et al. (30). Over a 20-year period (from ages 35–40 up to ages 55–60), Timio and colleagues closely observed cardiovascular and other parameters in 144 white Italian nuns in comparison with 133 control laywomen of the same ethnic background. The two groups differed in psychosocial environment (social isolation, meditation, and silence dominated the nunnery life style) but were similar in age and body weight and mass, as well as in family history of hypertension and daily salt intake (8 to 9 g sodium chloride). Plasma cholesterol and triglyceride levels were slightly, but not significantly, higher in the group of nuns. While the control group showed age-related increases in systolic and diastolic pressures typical of Western societies, both systolic and diastolic pressure stayed constant over the 20-year period in the group of nuns. The authors stressed that Western psychosocial influences on age-related increases of blood pressure must not be underestimated.

Whether menopause per se is a primary etiology for the development of hypertension is a complex question. Certainly the overall incidence of hypertension increases after the menopause, and certainly there are numerous physiological changes that occur in a woman's total health and cardiovascular system with aging and the cessation of ovarian production of estradiol and progesterone. This menopausal endocrine milieu may impact to some extent on a woman's polygenetically transferred predisposition to hypertension. Along with long-term influences of her psychosocial environment, declining levels of physical activity, increases in body-fat composition, and alterations in dietary and salt intake may facilitate or precipitate long-term cardiovascular structural adaptation and a gradual "structural upward resetting" (31) of the heart, vessels, and barostat mechanisms leading to hypertension.

The role of the gynecologist in the primary health care of the aging women is one of prevention and early detection of disease, and to insure that the patient has timely referrals for serious disorders that are beyond the scope of their practices. The detection of early hypertension and signs or symptoms of cardiac disease are vital issues in the ongoing care of the aging woman.

REFERENCES

1. Cummings SR, Black DM, Rubin SM. Lifetime risks of hip, Colles, or vertebral fracture and coronary heart disease among white postmenopausal women. Arch Intern Med 1989; 149:2445–2448.

2. Sigurdsson JA. High blood pressure in women: A cross-sectional and a longitudinal follow-up study. Acta Med Scand 1983; 669 (suppl):1–39.
3. Valkenburg HA, Hofman A, Klein F, et al. Een epidemiologisch onderzoek naar risico-indicatoren voor hart- en vaatziekten (EPOZ). I. Bloeddruk, serumcholesterolgehalte, Queteletindex en rookgewoonten in een open bevolking van vijf jaar en ouder. Ned T Geneesk 1980; 124:183–189.
4. Miall WE, Lovell HG. Relation between change of blood pressure and age. Br Med J 1977; 2:660–664.
5. Harlan WR, Hull AL, Schmouder RL, et al. Blood pressure and nutrition in adults: the National Health and Nutrition Examination Survey. Am J Epidemiol 1984; 120:17–28.
6. Landahl S, Bengtsson C, Sigurdsson JA, et al. Age-related changes in blood pressure. Hypertension 1986; 8:1044–1049.
7. Roberts JM. Oestrogens and hypertension. In: Biglieri EG, Schambelan M, eds. Clinics in Endocrinology and Metabolism. Philadelphia: WB Saunders, 1981:489–512.
8. Wilson PWF, Garrison RJ, Castelli WP. Postmenopausal estrogen use, cigarette smoking, and cardiovascular morbidity in women over 50: The Framingham Study. N Engl J Med 1985; 313:1038–1043.
9. Gordon T, Kannel WB, Hjortland MC, McNamara PM. Menopause and coronary heart disease: The Framingham study. Ann Intern Med 1978; 89:157–161.
10. Greenberg G, Imeson JD, Thompson SG, Meade TW. Blood pressure and the menstrual cycle. Br J Obstet Gynecol 1985; 92:1010–1014.
11. Casslen B. Blood pressure alter during the normal menstrual cycle. Br J Obstet Gynecol 1986; 93:523–526.
12. Lind T, Cameron EC, Hunter WM, et al. A prospective controlled trial of six forms of hormone replacement therapy given to postmenopausal women. Br J Obstet Gynecol 1979; 86(suppl 3):1–29.
13. Barrett-Connor E, Brown WV, Turner J, et al. Heart disease risk factors and hormone use in postmenopausal women. JAMA 1979; 241:2167–2169.
14. Kloosterboer HJ, van Wayjen RGA, van den Ende A. Effects of the oral contraceptive combination 0.150 mg desogestrel+0.020 mg ethinylestradiol on serum lipids including the HDL subfractions. Acta Obstet Gynecol Scand Suppl 1987; 144:33–36.

15. Kloosterboer HJ, van Wayjen RGA, van den Ende A. Effects of three low-dose oral contraceptive combinations on sex hormone binding globulin, corticosteroid binding globulin and antithrombin III activity in healthy women: two monophasic desogestrel combinations (containing 0.020 or 0.030 mg ethinylestradiol) and one triphasic levonorgestrel combination. Acta Obstet Gynecol Scand Suppl 1987; 144:41–44.

16. Adams MR, Clarkson TB, Koritnik DR, Nash H. Contraceptive steroids and coronary artery atherosclerosis in cynomolgus macaques. Fertil Steril 1987; 47:1010–1018.

17. Adams MR, Clarkson TB, Shively CA, et al. Oral contraceptives, lipoproteins and atherosclerosis. Am J Obstet Gynecol 1990;163: 1388–1393.

18. Lammers P, Atsma WJ. Metabolic effects of a new low-dose oral contraceptive containing 20 mcg ethinyloestradiol. Organorama 1990; 27(2):3–5.

19. Lobo RA. Cardiovascular implications of estrogen replacement therapy. Obstet Gynecol 1990; 75(suppl):18S–25S, 31S–35S.

20. PEPI Trial.

21. Messerli FH, Garavaglia GE, Schmieder RE, et al. Disparate cardiovascular findings in men and women with essential hypertension. Ann Intern Med 1987; 107:158–161.

22. Nachtigall LE. Cardiovascular disease and hypertension in older women. Obstet Gynecol Clin North Am 1987; 14:89–105.

23. Taylor RD, Corcoran AC, Page IH. Menopausal hypertension: a critical study. Am J Med Sci 1947; 213:475–476.

24. Weiss NS. Relationship of menopause to serum cholesterol and arterial blood pressure: the United States Health Examination Survey of Adults. Am J Epidemiol 1972; 96:237–241.

25. Cornoni-Huntley J, Harlan WR, Leaverton PE. Blood pressure in adolescence: the United States Health Examination Survey. Hypertension 1979; 1:559–566.

26. Reisen E, Abel R, Modan M, et al. Effect of weight loss without salt restriction on the reduction of blood pressure in overweight hypertensive patients. N Engl J Med 1978; 298:1–6.

27. Wade GN, Gray JM. Gonadal effects on food intake and adiposity: a metabolic hypothesis. Physiol Behav 1979; 22:583–593.

28. van Beresteijn ECLH, Riedstra M, van der Wel A, et al. Habitual dietary calcium intake and blood pressure change around the menopause: a longitudinal study. Int J Epidemiol 1992; 21:683–689.

29. Wu Z, Wu X, Zhang Y. Relationship of menopausal status and sex hormones to serum lipids and blood pressure. Int J Epidemiol 1990; 19:297–302.
30. Timio M, Verdecchia P, Venanzi S, et al. Age and blood pressure changes: a 20-year follow-up study in nuns in a secluded order. Hypertension 1988; 12:457–461.
31. Folkow B. The pathophysiology of hypertension: Differences between young and elderly patients. Drugs 1993; 46:3–7.

13

Antihypertensive Therapy in Hypertensive Postmenopausal Women

Thorsten Fischer and Roland E. Schmieder

University of Erlangen/Nuernberg
Klinikum Nuernberg
Nuernberg, Germany

Franz C. Aepfelbacher and Franz H. Messerli

Ochsner Clinic and
Alton Ochsner Medical Foundation
New Orleans, Louisiana

I. OVERVIEW

Hypertension is one of the most important risk factors for cardio-vascular morbidity and mortality, requiring rigorous pharmaco-logical therapy if resistant to nonpharmacological interventions. The four first-line drug classes that are used for antihypertensive treatment are: angiotensin-converting enzyme (ACE) inhibitors, calcium antagonists, beta-blockers, and diuretics. They all reduce blood pressure to a similar extent, but an individualized approach is recommended with respect to concomitant cardiovascular risk factors and diseases. General guidelines for the treatment of postmenopausal women have been published by the Joint National Committee (5,6) and the German Hypertension Liga (4); however, more specific therapeutic guidelines do not exist for these patients. In this regard it is important to realize that gender-related differences of hypertensive disease exist. At similar levels of blood pressure, left ventricular hypertrophy is more frequently seen in women than in men. If left ventricular hypertrophy is present in a female hypertensive patient, those drug classes known to reduce left ventricular hypertrophy should be preferred. ACE inhibitors effectively reduce left ventricular hypertrophy, making it a good choice for the treatment of arterial hypertension with coexisting left ventricular hypertrophy. Thiazide diuretics are recommended in postmenopausal women with increased risk of osteoporosis-related complications due to a beneficial effect on urinary loss of calcium.

In addition, considering the specific hemodynamic profile of female hypertensives and the potential side effects of pharmacological treatment, risks of antihypertensive medication can be limited. Thus, not only is the cardiovascular risk expected to decrease by treating hypertension, but the patient's quality of life may be improved as well.

II. INTRODUCTION

Hypertension is a major risk factor of cardiovascular morbidity and mortality, leading to sudden cardiac death, myocardial infarction, congestive heart failure, and cerebral ischemia (20). It is estimated that the risk of myocardial infarction can be reduced by 2–3% for each 1–mm Hg reduction of diastolic blood pressure (82). A meta-analysis in 43,000 patients with mild essential hypertension further revealed that pharmacological reduction of diastolic blood pressure by 5 to 6 mm Hg over 5 years reduces the incidence of stroke by 42% and of myocardial infarction by nearly 14% (18). (The importance of these data influences the current treatment strategies for arterial hypertension. As a consequence, it was recommended that blood pressure be kept below 90 mm Hg.) Nonpharmacological interventions, including moderate sodium restriction, reduced alcohol intake, weight loss, and physical exercise, are the primary steps to control high blood pressure, independent of the gender of the hypertensives.

This chapter focuses on pharmacological antihypertensive treatment in postmenopausal women. In particular, it considers the question of whether *specific* recommendations for treatment of postmenopausal women can be made.

III. PRETREATMENT CONSIDERATIONS

1. Nearly 50% of all individuals suffering from high blood pressure are not aware of their disease. Therefore, gaining access to these subjects is a most challenging issue in primary prevention. Patients with mild to moderate arterial hypertension are mostly asymptomatic. The fact that postmenopausal women contact their gynecologists relatively often (for cancer screening or osteoporosis-induced or climacteric complaints)—more often than men of the same age see their doctors—offers an opportunity that unfortunately is not used adequately to screen for high blood pressure.

2. In the diagnosis and treatment of arterial hypertension, it is essential to apply correct techniques for measurement of blood pressure. Twenty-four-hour ambulatory blood-pressure monitoring has been shown to reflect hypertensive target-organ damage more accurately than casual blood-pressure measurements. Furthermore, for detection of white-coat hypertension (elevated values of casual blood pressure but normal ambulatory blood pressure) and reversed white-coat hypertension (normal casual blood pressure but elevated ambulatory blood pressure), physicians should preferentially use methods that allow the measurement of blood pressure over a longer period of time under natural conditions, such as self-measurement of blood pressure and ambulatory blood-pressure measurements (72,73).

3. After the diagnosis of arterial hypertension has been

established, the next step in the patient's care is to determine the best individualized therapeutic regimen (nonpharmacological versus pharmacological therapy, selection of antihypertensive agent), then to keep control of the patient's compliance with the chosen therapy. This is not the easiest part, as it is known that as many as 50% of patients who start on antihypertensive therapy will drop out within 1 year. Only a minority of patients, particularly those who are well informed about their disease, remain under the physician's control (41).

4. Before antihypertensive drug therapy is begun, other risk factors of cardiovascular diseases—such as obesity, diabetes mellitus, and hyperlipidemia—should be screened for, and treated, if necessary. Coexistence of other cardiovascular risk factors makes antihypertensive therapy even more important since the cardiovascular risks increase exponentially if hypertension is accompanied by diabetes mellitus and the other risk factors mentioned above (46).

There is a close association between obesity and high blood pressure and related heart diseases. Interestingly, it seems that rigorous weight reduction is more effective in men than in women with regard to lowering blood pressure (36). There is no doubt, however, that weight reduction can reduce the risk of high blood pressure and myocardial infarction in men and in women.

To lower the cardiovascular risk, treatment of diabetes mellitus is similarly important. The cardiovascular risk seems to be sex-specific. Age-adjusted mortality rates for coronary heart disease are three to seven times higher among diabetic women than among nondiabetic women. In comparison, the sex-specific risk for diabetic men is "only" two to three times higher than for nondiabetics (53). Therapeutic interventions will limit these life-threatening complications of diabetes mellitus if therapy is started without delay.

Compared to men of the same age, premenopausal women have higher HDL and lower LDL cholesterol levels. With the onset of menopause, however, serum levels of total cholesterol, LDL cholesterol, apolipoprotein A1, apolipoprotein B, and tri-glyceride increase significantly, which leads to an enormous increase in coronary atherosclerosis, particularly if risk factors such as hypertension or smoking are present (16,28,59). Once hyperlipidemia is diagnosed, it should be treated with diet and/or lipid-lowering drugs. In the case of concomitant hypertension, it should be taken into consideration that two of the first-choice antihypertensive agents—diuretics and beta-blockers—may induce and/or aggravate hyperlipidemia to some extent, and this may occur even after years of therapy.

5. The choice of an antihypertensive agent must be based on the individual history of each patient, age, body weight, and presence or absence of coexisting cardiovascular risk factors and concomitant diseases. Blood pressure needs to be "normalized" when signs of hypertensive organ damage are present, such as congestive heart failure, left ventricular hypertrophy, renal involvement (reduced creatinine clearance or microalbuminuria), or hypertensive retinopathy. The effect of antihypertensive treatment has been investigated in multiple studies, and a benefit was seen even in patients with mild essential hypertension (90 to 110 mm Hg of diastolic blood pressure) (7,8). A working party of the British Hypertension Society suggested, in accordance with recommendations of other hypertension study groups, that in the elderly a sustained arterial systolic pressure of greater than 160 mm Hg or a sustained diastolic pressure of greater than 90 mm Hg, or both, should be treated (80).

IV. DRUG THERAPY

A. General Aspects

Nowadays a variety of antihypertensive drugs are available. They differ from one another in their pharmacodynamic profile, mode of action, pharmacokinetics, and side effects. The aim of these drugs—namely, to effectively lower high blood pressure with no or few side effects—is best achieved by an individualized approach. In addition to diuretics and beta-blockers, substances that have been used for a long time in the treatment of arterial hypertension, newer classes such as calcium antagonists and ACE inhibitors have been introduced in the last decade. At present, these four drug classes are recommended for initial antihypertensive drug treatment. Table 1 summarizes important aspects in the selection of an appropriate antihypertensive medication.

Favorable effects of calcium antagonists and ACE inhibitors are characterized by neutrality in lipid and glucose metabolism. Adverse effects of glucose and lipid metabolism may increase the risk of coronary artery disease, thereby offsetting the cardioprotective antihypertensive effects (35). ACE inhibitors have evolved as being especially effective in reducing left ventricular hypertrophy as well as vascular hypertrophy (50,56,57,65).

B. Angiotensin-Converting Enzyme Inhibitors

1. Description

Angiotensin-converting enzyme inhibitors reduce the synthesis of angiotensin I to angiotensin II, thereby inhibiting angiotensin II–induced vasoconstriction. In addition, they induce a decrease in aldosterone secretion, leading to an increased natriuresis (30). In contrast to other vasodilators (dihydralazine, minoxidil), ACE inhibitors do not activate the sympathetic nervous system indicated by the lack of reflexive tachycardia. Aside from their effects on the renin-angiotensin-aldosterone system, ACE inhibitors decrease the inactivation of bradykinin, which results in an increase of vasodilatory prostaglandins (26). Thus, ACE inhibitors lower blood pressure by reducing total peripheral resistance without significantly affecting heart rate or cardiac output (14,30,32, 70,84,87). Furthermore, these substances seem to increase coronary perfusion by local blockade of angiotensin II.

ACE inhibitors are particularly useful for patients who have developed systolic ventricular dysfunction or even congestive heart failure. Several prospective studies have documented that ACE inhibitors reduce total cardiovascular mortality in patients with reduced systolic function or incipient or severe congestive heart failure (2). In addition to lowering the load of the left ventricle, ACE inhibitors also counteract the sympathetic ner-

Table 1 Checklist of Limitations on Use of Hypotensive Drugs in Patients with a Second Condition

	ACE inhibitors	Calcium antagonists	Beta-blockers	Diuretics
Antihypertensive efficiency (high response rate and low side effects)	Yes	Yes	Yes	Yes
Preferential use in menopause (hemodynamic viewpoint)	Yes	Yes	With reservation	With reservation
Prove of reduction in cardiovascular mortality and morbidity (primary prevention)	Not yet[a]	No	Yes	Yes
Impairment of lipid metabolism	No	No	Yes	Yes
Reduction of left ventricular hypertrophy in excess of afterload reduction	Yes	Probably	No	No
Nephroprotective properties	Yes	Probably	No	No
Coexisting disease				
Diabetes mellitus	Yes	Yes	Care needed[b]	Care needed[c]
Gout	Yes	Yes	Yes	No
Ischemic heart disease	Yes	Yes	Yes	Yes
Heart failure	Yes	Care needed[d]	No	Yes
Asthma	Yes	Yes	No	Yes
Peripheral vascular disease	Care needed	Yes	Care needed	Yes
Renal artery stenosis	No	Yes[d]	Yes	Yes

Based on recommendations of the British Hypertension Society (80) and Schmieder et al. (78).

[a] ACE inhibitors for primary prevention are under investigations (61).

[b] Beta-blockers should be used with care in diabetes because awareness of insulin hypoglycemia may be dulled. In non-insulin-dependent disease beta-blockers may worsen glucose tolerance and exacerbate the deranged lipid profile.

[c] Diuretics may exacerbate diabetes.

[d] Care is needed when using calcium antagonists, particularly verapamil and diltiazem, in heart failure.

Table 2 Angiotensin-Converting Enzyme
Inhibitors

Drug	Usual dose (mg/d)	24-hr blood-pressure control with once-daily dosage
Benazepril	10–40	Yes
Captopril	12.5–150	No
Cilazapril	2.5–5	Yes
Enalapril	2.5–40	Yes
Fosinopril	10–40	Yes
Lisinopril	5–40	Yes
Perindopril	1–16	Yes
Quinapril	5–80	No
Ramipril	1.25–20	Yes
Spirapril	12.5–50	Yes

Hemodynamic mechanism: peripheral vasodilation.
Side effects: cough, impairment of renal function, hypotension (especially in combination with diuretics), hyperkalemia (in combination with renal insufficiency or potassium-sparing agents), angioneurotic edema, leukopenia.
Contraindications: pregnancy, bilateral renal artery stenosis, or renal artery stenosis (if only one function).
Cautions: renal insufficiency, high potassium levels, renovascular disease (i.e., intrarenal artery stenosis).

vous system and the renin-angiotensin-aldosterone system, both of which are stimulated in congestive heart failure. Furthermore, ACE inhibitors lead to a regression of left ventricular hypertrophy, thereby reducing the risk of cardiac sudden death and myocardial infarction (24). The increase of left ventricular mass correlates with aging and the female sex and is therefore seen more frequently in elderly women (55).

Besides the cardioprotective effects, ACE inhibitors also protect against cerebrovascular and renal damage due to arterial hypertension. Renal blood flow is increased by ACE inhibitors but intraglomerular pressure is reduced simultaneously (90). This intraglomerular hemodynamic effect prevents and at least delays the development of glomerulosclerosis in patients with arterial hypertension and reduced kidney function. An increase of renal perfusion and glomerular filtration was detected after starting antihypertensive therapy with ACE inhibitors (11,12, 39,40,52,76,88).

Because of the decrease in the activity of the renin-angiotensin-aldosterone system with increasing age, the efficacy of ACE inhibitors in the elderly has been controversial. Nevertheless, it has been demonstrated that they decrease arterial blood pressure equally effectively in young and elderly patients (44). ACE inhibitors have been well accepted by physicians and patients, not only because of their clinical efficiency, but also because of the remarkably few side effects and the improvement in quality of life.

1. Side Effects and Contraindications

ACE inhibitors are well tolerated, with only few side effects that are not influenced by age (77). The most frequent ACE-inhibitor-associated side effect is cough (19). Approximately 2 to 10% of all hypertensive patients receiving ACE inhibitors develop a drug-related cough, which occurs more frequently in women (31). The underlying mechanism is attributed to accumulation of bradykinin; consequently, it is not surprising that the selective angiotensin II receptor blockers do not produce this side effect.

More important is the impairment of renal function with ACE-inhibitor therapy in patients with bilateral artery stenosis. This is more common in the elderly patient.

As a measure of precaution, serum creatinine and serum potassium should be controlled after approximately 1 week. If serum potassium exceeds normal limits (most frequently in patients with renal insufficiency and/or potassium-sparing diuretics) or serum creatinine increases by more than 40%, discontinuation of ACE-inhibitor medication is required, and, in cases of excessive increases of serum creatinine, diagnostic tests for renal artery stenosis are indicated. The initial dose of ACE inhibitors should be reduced by half for the first 3 days in patients on diuretics, with hypovolemia, or with high plasma renin levels, as serious hypotension may occur under these circumstances (13,21,

37). A significant relationship between age and side effects of ACE inhibitors has not been described. Although counterregulation to hypotension is reduced in the elderly (impaired baroreceptor function), the incidence of hypotension under ACE-inhibitor therapy is not increased if the abovementioned circumstances are considered.

Angioneurotic edema related to ACE inhibitors is very rare; however, it may be serious if it occurs (19,45).

C. Calcium Antagonists

1. Description

Another class of substances that has become well accepted in the treatment of hypertension are calcium antagonists. The first generation of calcium antagonists include nifedipine, verapamil, and diltiazem, which seem to be comparable with respect to their blood-pressure-lowering properties. The second generation in-

Table 3 Calcium Antagonists

Drug	Usual dose (mg/d)	24-hr blood-pressure control with once-daily dosage	Slow-release available?
Diltiazem SR/ER	90–360	No	Yes
Verapamil/RR	80–480	No	Yes
Amlodipine	2.5–10	Yes	Unnecessary
Felodipine	5–20	Yes	Yes
Isradipine/SR	2.5–10	No	Yes
Nicardipine	60–120	No	—
Nifedipine	30–120	No	Yes
Nitrendipine	5–40	Yes	—

Hemodynamic mechanism: peripheral vasodilation.
Side effects: headache, flush, postural hypotension, peripheral edema, nocturia, hepatic toxicity (very rarely).
Contraindications: atrioventricular block (caution needed in combination with beta-blocker), and left ventricular dysfunction (only for diltiazem and verapamil).
Cautions: dihydropyridines are more potent peripheral vasodilators than diltiazem and verapamil and may cause more dizziness, peripheral edema, headache, and tachycardia.

cludes amlodipine, felodipine, isradipine, and nicardipine, which all require only once-a-day medication due to a prolonged half-life of slow-release forms.

These compounds inhibit calcium entry into cardiac and smooth-muscle cells through blockade of voltage-dependent channels. They interfere with calcium-dependent contractions of vascular smooth muscle, thereby leading to direct vasodilatation (58). Through the activation of arterial baroreflex mechanisms, cardiac sympathetic activity is augmented, leading to an increased heart rate (69) in calcium antagonists of the nifedipine type. In contrast, the direct AV-node-blocking effect of diltiazem and verapamil counteracts any reflex-induced increase in cardiac sympathetic activity. In addition, calcium antagonists block receptor-operated channels, including alpha-adrenoreceptors and angiotensin II receptors, that support calcium flux into the cells (85).

Calcium antagonists reduce left ventricular hypertrophy to a somewhat smaller extent than ACE inhibitors, but maintain or even increase blood flow of the coronary circulation and renal perfusion similar to the extent observed after ACE inhibition (9). Calcium channel blockers are particularly effective in elderly patients, exhibiting only few side effects (10,27,74). Due to this pharmacological profile they are very useful for postmenopausal hypertensive women. Some authors have reported that the anti-hypertensive effect of calcium antagonists correlates with age (17), but this issue remains controversial.

Calcium antagonists have been found to be effective alone or in combination with other antihypertensive drugs. As drugs of first choice they lower mild to moderate hypertensive pressure levels in the majority of patients to an extent similar to that documented for the other three first-line drugs (54).

2. Side Effects and Contraindications

Serious side effects of calcium antagonists are rare. Ankle edema, headaches, or flushing, however, are relatively common due to their vasodilatory action. In menopausal women with left ventricular dysfunction or conduction disorders, verapamil and diltiazem should be used cautiously because of their negative chronotropic and inotropic effects (60,62). In women who are predisposed to peripheral edema due to venous insufficiency, administration of the dihydropyridine–calcium antagonists frequently leads to pedal edema, whereas verapamil or diltiazem only rarely cause this side effect (49). Additional caution is required in treating elderly women prone to develop postural hypotension (62,67,68). In these cases, slow-dose titration may help to reduce these side effects. Very rarely, calcium channel blockers cause hepatic toxicity, eye discomfort, or nocturia (89).

D. Beta-Blockers

1. Description

Besides diuretics, beta-adrenergic receptor blockers have traditionally been the most popular drugs for treatment of arterial hypertension. Several disorders that occur more frequently in the elderly, such as congestive heart failure, peripheral vascular diseases, diabetes mellitus, hyperlipidemia, psychiatric disorders (e.g., depression), and chronic obstructive pulmonary disease, limit the use of beta-blockers as drugs of first choice in the treatment of essential hypertension. Nevertheless, beta-blockers are well-established drugs for the secondary prevention after myocardial infarction. Hence, in hypertensive patients who have had myocardial infarction and/or angina pectoris, beta-blockers should be prescribed preferentially as long as other contraindications do not exist. No differences between women and men have been seen in the cardioprotective effect.

Beta-blockers lower high blood pressure by decreasing cardiac output, renin release, and central sympathetic nervous activity (61). In contrast, total peripheral resistance was found to be increased even after long-term treatment, at rest, and, in particular, during stress due to a relative preponderance of alpha-receptor-mediated vasoconstriction. This unfavorable hemodynamic finding excludes the use of beta-blockers in patients with peripheral arterial disease.

Table 4   Beta-Blockers

Drug	Usual dose (mg/d)	24-hr blood-pressure control with once-daily dosage
Beta-blockers		
Acebutolol	200–1200	No
Atenolol	25–100	Yes
Betaxolol	5–40	Yes
Bisoprolol	5–20	Yes
Carteolol	2.5–10	Yes
Metoprolol	50–200	Yes
Nadolol	20–240	Yes
Penbutolol	20–80	Yes
Pindolol	10–60	No
Propranolol	40–240	No
Timolol	20–40	No
Alpha-beta blockers		
Labetalol	200–1200	Yes

Hemodynamic mechanism: reduction of cardiac output.
Side effects: bronchospasm, hypocglycemia, glucose intolerance, hypertri-glyceridemia, HDL cholesterol reduction, AV block.
Contraindications: chronic obstructive lung disease, peripheral vascular disease, cardiac insufficiency.
Cautions: coronary spasm, insulin-requiring diabetes.

2.   Side Effects and Contraindications

Some studies suggest that beta-blockers are particularly effective in the treatment of hypertensive individuals with high renin levels and are less effective in elderly patients since plasma renin activity declines with age (17,66,15,86). Indeed, beta-blockers have more favorable results in young individuals than in elderly hypertensives. Elderly patients who are on beta-blocker therapy have more side effects together with a lower drug toleration than younger patients treated with these agents. In postmenopausal women with decreased left ventricular systolic function and/or bradycardia, the negative inotropic and chronotropic effects of beta-blockers are relative contraindications for therapy with those drugs, which at least require specific attention when used for blood-pressure control.

Contraindications for beta-blockers are chronic obstructive pulmonary disease, peripheral vascular disease, heart failure, and AV block grade II or III.

E. Diuretics

1. Description

Despite the introduction of calcium antagonists and ACE inhibitors into therapy, diuretics are still very popular drugs for the treatment of arterial hypertension. Diuretics are effective in lowering systolic and diastolic blood pressure, particularly in hypertensive elderly individuals (29,43,63) and have been shown to reduce cardiovascular mortality in primary prevention. The initial reduction of blood pressure is achieved by lowering total blood volume through the inhibition of sodium and chloride cotransport across the tubular luminal membrane in the kidney. Rarely, a transient fall in cardiac output is observed. However, with prolonged treatment, the major hemodynamic effect of diuretics is a decrease in total peripheral resistance with normal blood volume and cardiac output.

Due to their potassium-losing properties, thiazides are usually combined with potassium-sparing agents, such as amiloride, triamterene, and, less frequently, spironolactone. These combinations proved to be very useful because of their synergistic effect in natriuresis and their antagonistic effect in potassium loss. The aldrosterone-antagonist spironolactone is also very effective in natriuresis, but side effects—such as gynecomastia—limit its use. More potent diuretics, e.g., ethacrynic acid, furosemide, and bumetanide, which act on the ascending thick limb of Henle's loop, are not used for chronic treatment of arterial hypertension because of their rapid and short action and potentially serious side effects (hypokalemia).

Diuretics are preferentially used in hypertensive patients with concomitant edema and congestive heart failure or in other circumstances with volume overload (but not in pregnancy-induced hypertension, because of a decrease in uteroplacental blood flow).

Table 5 Diuretics

Drug	Usual dose (mg/d)	24-hr blood-pressure control with once-daily dosage
Thiazides		
Bendroflumethiazide	2.5–5	Yes
Benzthiazide	12.5–50	Yes
Chlorothiazide	125–500	No
Chlorthalidone	12.5–50	Yes
Cyclothiazide	1–2	Yes
Hydrochlorthiazide	12.5–50	Yes
Hydroflumetiazide	12.5–50	Yes
Indapamide	2.5–5	Yes
Methyclothiazide	2.5–5	Yes
Metolazone	0.5–5	Yes
Polythiazide	1–4	Yes
Quinethazone	25–100	Yes
Trichlormethiazide	1–4	Yes
Loop diuretics		
Bumetanide	0.5–5	No
Ethacrync acid	25–100	No
Furosemide	20–320	No
Torasemide	10–200	Yes
Potasium-sparing agents		
Amiloride	5–10	Yes
Spironolactone	25–100	Yes
Triamterene	50–100	Yes

Hemodynamic mechanism: initial volume decrease, peripheral vasodilatation.
Side effects: hypokalemia (influencing arrhythmias in hypertensives and in combination with digitalis), glucose intolerance, hypercholesterolemia, hyperuricemia.
Contraindications: pre-existing hypovolemia.
Cautions: hypokalemia, diabetes mellitus, pretreated with digitalis, gout.

2. Side Effects and Contraindications

Hypokalemia is probably the most serious side effect of diuretic therapy that may be associated with an increased incidence of arrhythmias (3,38,42). This is of special importance for older patients because so many have coronary heart disease and are therefore taking digitalis medication. It has been reported that up to 30% of patients on diuretics develop hypokalemia or hypomagnesemia (48). Indeed, a subgroup of hypertensives with ECG abnormalities at baseline who were on diuretics had an increased incidence of cardiac sudden death in comparison with controls receiving placebo (3). An exaggerated ventricular ectopy mediated by hypokalemia seemed to be responsible for these findings, suggesting that thiazide diuretics should be used only in combination with potassium-sparing agents in this patient group. In addition, electrolyte impairment is less commonly observed if diuretics are given at lower doses and, therefore, both low-dose treatment and combination with a potassium-sparing component are now recommended to counteract the side effects of hypokalemia and/or hypomagnesemia.

The impact of diuretics on calcium metabolism is of particular significance for postmenopausal women. Loop diuretics and thiazides (hydrochlorothiazide and chlorthalidone), but not bendrofluazide, reduce tubular calcium absorption (25,33,34). This effect might lead to an increase of serum calcium, thereby suppressing the secretion of parathyroid hormone. Clinical studies have shown that long-term therapy with diuretics in the elderly correlates with a decrease in hip fractures (51) and long-term thiazide therapy reduces the urinary loss of calcium (64,83). Therefore, in postmenopausal women for whom supplementation of calcium is recommended, diuretics might be considered the first choice of antihypertensive drugs.

Recent studies have demonstrated a positive effect of estrogen replacement therapy on calcium metabolism, especially when estrogen deficiency is present at the menopause. Furthermore, risk can also be reduced through nutrition (intake of milk products), supplementation of calcium, and physical exercise (1,23,79).

F.   Choice of Drug

It is our opinion that diuretics, beta-blockers, calcium antagonists, and ACE inhibitors are drugs of first choice in the treatment of high blood pressure. Section of a particular drug should follow an individualized strategy (78).

When choosing the appropriate antihypertensive medication, the individual history of a patient, the cardiovascular risk-factor profile, concomitant diseases, and therapeutic costs must be considered. These considerations together with the physician's own experience will allow every patient to be treated effectively and safely.

Due to the increase of blood pressure with the onset of menopause, high blood pressure is often first diagnosed at this time. The question of when to start pharmacological therapy in those newly diagnosed hypertensive women has always been, and probably will remain, a controversial issue. However, if high blood-pressure levels are measured several times and nonpharmacological regimens are ineffective, pharmacological treatment should be initiated as soon as possible, particularly if other cardiovascular risk factors or symptoms of hypertension-related damage to the heart (left ventricular hypertrophy), kidneys (albuminuria), or arteries (fundoscopic changes) are present. The four drug classes characterized above are currently recommended as first-line agents for antihypertensive therapy (6). However, these recommendations vary with time (JNC 1988 versus JNC 1993) (5,6) and from country to country (JNC 1993 USA versus Hypertension Liga Germany 1994) (3,4). In 1988, the JNC recommended the use of diuretics, beta-blockers, calcium antagonists, and ACE inhibitors as first-line antihypertensive drugs. However, these recommendations have changed over time and in 1993 the JNC advised that diuretics and beta-blockers be used preferentially.

The decision as to which drug class will initially be prescribed is influenced by a physician's individual experience. When the decision has been made to treat elevated arterial blood pressure, only one antihypertensive drug should be used in initial treatment. If monotherapy does not prove effective, the initial drug should be stopped and a new drug class should be considered (sequential therapy). It can be expected that in 50 to 60% of all treated patients, arterial blood pressure is not adequately controlled or side effects are not acceptable. If blood-pressure control is not sufficient with the second monotherapy, a combination should be used of two or more antihypertensive drugs that act differently. Combination therapy may increase the antihypertensive effects and lessen the degree of side effects of each single drug since lower doses can be used.

The hemodynamic changes that occur around menopause may induce high blood pressure in previously normotensive women. Premenopausal women seem to be protected against these changes because of their greater estrogen production. In patients with hypertension before menopause, effective antihypertensive treatment should not be altered just because of menopause. If therapy is not sufficient, the drug dosage should be increased or an additional drug class added. Clearly, the general guidelines for the treatment of hypertension—JNC 1988, JNC 1993, and German Liga 1994 (3,5,6)—are also valid for women around or after menopause.

Since many women undergo hysterectomy with or without oophorectomy, the influence of such a surgical intervention on blood pressure must be considered. It is known that physiological estrogen synthesis in these women can significantly decrease after a hysterectomy even without oophorectomy. Patients who do not receive adequate hormone substitution are affected by early "artificial" menopause with an increased risk for coronary disease and hypertension (22,81). Data from the Framingham Study have shown that the cardiovascular risk associated with early surgically induced menopause is even higher than with naturally occurring menopause (47). Therefore, consequent antihypertensive drug treatment is particularly important in this group of women to reduce cardiovascular morbidity and mortality.

Women after menopause may experience a change in the quality of life because of a variety of cofactors, such as change in social interaction, coexisting climacteric complaints, depression, or increase of cancer. Additional negative effects resulting from failed antihypertensive therapy should therefore be avoided. An important consideration is the effect of antihypertensive therapy on sexual function. ACE inhibitors and, to a lesser extent, calcium antagonists are known to potentially impair sexual function in men, but their effects on sexual function in women have not been adequately investigated.

Osteoporosis, and its complications, is one of the most important disorders in postmenopausal women. Bone mass, a useful predictor of fracture risk, is significantly lower in women than in men of the same age. Of patients with osteoporosis-related fractures, those with hip fractures have the highest incidence of morbidity, with a 1-year mortality of up to 30% (79). Thiazide diuretics are the only class of antihypertensive drugs that have a protective effect on the incidence of hip fractures. This could not be demonstrated for other diuretics (75).

In an unselected population, such as the Framingham cohort, echocardiographic studies showed a higher prevalence of left ventricular hypertrophy in women (19%) than in men (16%) (55). The incidence of left ventricular mass correlates with aging; it increases from 5% in women under the age of 30 to 49% in women aged 70 years or older (versus an increase from 8% to 33% in men of the same ages). In selected hypertensive patients, up to 48% were reported to have echocardiographic left ventricular hypertrophy. Due to the increased cardiovascular risk (sudden death, myocardial infarction, stroke) in patients with left ventricular hypertrophy as compared to patients without left ventricular hypertrophy (24), the effect of antihypertensive drug therapy on left ventricular mass has to be considered. ACE inhibitors have been shown to reduce left ventricular hypertrophy most effectively, making it a good choice for the treatment of arterial hypertension in postmenopausal women with coexisting left ventricular hypertrophy.

In conclusion, decisions in antihypertensive therapy are influenced by different underlying hemodynamic mechanisms and side effects of the chosen drugs. The four first-choice antihypertensive drug classes—angiotensin-converting enzyme inhibitors, calcium antagonists, beta-blockers, and diuretics—are effective in reducing arterial hypertension, thereby reducing hypertension-associated morbidity and mortality.

REFERENCES

1. Consensus Development Conference. Diagnosis, prophylaxis, and treatment of osteoporosis. Am J Med 1993; 94:646–650.
2. Consensus Study Trial Group. Effects of enalapril on mortality in severe congestive heart failure: Results of the North Scandinavian enalapril survival study. N Engl J Med 1987; 316:1429–1435.
3. Medical Research Council Working Party on Mild to Moderate Hypertension. Ventricular extrasystoles during thiazide treatment: Study of MRC Mild Hypertension Trial. Br Med J 1983; 287:1249–1253.
4. Recommendations of the German Hypertension Liga, Heidelberg, 1994.
5. The Fifth Report of the Joint National Committee on Detection, Evaluation and Treatment of High Blood Pressure. NIH publication 93-1088. Bethesda, MD: National Institutes of Health, 1993: 11–30.
6. The 1988 Joint National Committee. The 1988 report of the Joint National Committee on Detection, Evaluation, and Treatment of High Blood Pressure. Arch Intern Med 1988; 148:1023–1038.
7. The Management Committee. Initial results of the Australian Therapeutic Trial in mild hypertension. Clin Sci 1979; 57:449–452.
8. The Cooperative Group. Five year findings of the hypertension detection and follow-up program. JAMA 1979; 213:2562–2571.
9. Amodeo C, Kobrin I, Ventura HO. Immediate and short term hemodynamic effects of diltiazem in patients with hypertension. Circulation 1986; 73:108–113.
10. Abernethy DR, Schwartz JB, Luchi R, Snoe E. Verapamil pharmacodynamics and disposition in young and elderly hypertensive patients: altered electrocardiographic and hypotensive responses. Ann Intern Med 1986; 105:329–336.
11. Bauer JH. Effects of enalapril alone, and in combination with hydrothiazide, on renin-angiotensin-aldosterone, renal function, salt and water excretion, and body fluid composition. Am J Kidney Dis 1985; 6:222–232.
12. Bauer JH, Reams P. Renal protective effect of strict blood pressure control with enalapril therapy. Arch Intern Med 1987; 147:1397–1400.
13. Benett PR, Cairns SA. Captopril, diarrhoea and hypotension. Lancet 1985; i:1105.

14. Brunner HR. Effects of angiotensin converting enzyme inhibition: a clinical point of view. J Cardiovasc Pharmacol 1985; 7(suppl 4): 73–81.

15. Bertel O, Buhler FR, Kiowski W, Lutold BE. Decreased beta-adrenoreceptor responsiveness as related to age, blood pressure and plasma catecholamines in patients with essential hypertension. Hypertension 1980; 2:130–138.

16. Bonithon-Koop C, Scarabin Y, Darne B, Malmejac A, Guize L. Menopause related changes in lipoproteins and some other cardiovascular risk factors. Int J Epidemiol 1990; 19:42–48.

17. Buhler FR, Boll P, Krowski W. Renin profiling to select antihypertensive baseline drugs. Am J Med 1984; 77:36–42.

18. Collins R, Peto R, MacMahon S, Herbert P, Fiebach H, Eberlein KA. Blood pressure, stroke and coronary heart disease. Part 2. Short term reductions in blood pressure: overview of randomized drug trials in their epidemiological context. Lancet 1990; 335:827–838.

19. Cooper WD, Sheldon D, Brown D. Postmarketing surveillance of enalapril: Experience in 11710 hypertensive patients in general practice. J R Coll Gen Pract 1987; 37:346.

20. Corrao TL, Becker RC, Ockene IS. Coronary heart disease risk factors in women. Cardiology 1990; 77(suppl 2):8–24.

21. Coulshed DJ, Davies SJ, Turney JH. Prolonged hypotension after fever during enalapril treatment. Lancet 1985; 2:222.

22. Cust P, Whitehead MI, Powles R, Hunter M, Milliken S. Consequences and treatment of ovarian failure after total body irradiation for leukaemia. Br Med J 1989; 299:1494–1497.

23. Dalsky GP, Stocke KS, Ehsani M, Slatopolsky E, Lee WC, Birge SJ. Weight bearing exercise training and lumber bone mineral content in postmenopausal women. Ann Intern Med 1988; 108:824–828.

24. Devereux RB, Casala PN, Savage DD, Laragh JH. Relation of left ventricular mass and geometry to morbidity and mortality in uncomplicated essential hypertension. Ann Intern Med 1991; 114: 345–352.

25. Donath A, Nordio S, Macagno F, Gatti R. The effect of hydrochlorthiazide on calcium and strontium transport in intestine and kidney. Helv Paediat Acta 1971; 25:293–300.

26. Douglas JG. Douglas JG. Subpressor infusions of angiotensin II after glomerular binding, prostaglandin E2, and cyclic AMP production. Hypertension 1987; 11(suppl 3):49–56.

27. Dzau BJ. Evolution of the clinical management of hypertension:

emerging role of "specific" vasodilators as initial therapy. Am J Med 1987; 82:36–43.

28. Fletcher AE, Bulpitt CJ. Epidemiological aspects of cardiovascular disease in the elderly. J Hypertension 1992; 10(suppl 2):51–58.

29. Freis ED. Age and antihypertensive drugs (hydrocholorothiazide, bendromethiazide, nadolol and captopril). Am J Cardiol 1988; 61:117–121.

30. Frohlich ED. Angiotensin converting enzyme: Present and future. Hypertension 1989; 13(suppl 1):125–130.

31. Fuller RW, Dixon CMS, Cuss FMC. Bradykinin induced bronchoconstriction in humans. Annu Rev Respir Dis 1987; 135:176.

32. Gomez HJ. The clinical pharmacology of lisinopril. J Cardiovasc Pharmacol 1987; 9(suppl 3):27–34.

33. Gursel E. Effects of diuretics on renal intestinal handling of calcium. NY State J Med 1970; 70:399–405.

34. Harrison AR, Ross GA. The effect of bendrofluozide on urinary and faecal calcium and phosphorus. Clin Sci 1986; 34:343–350.

35. Heyden S, Schneider KA, Fodor GJ. Failure to reduce cholesterol as explanation for the limited efficacy of antihypertensive treatment in the reduction of CHD. Klin Wochensch 1987; 65:828–832.

36. Higgins M, Kannel W, Garrison R, Pinsky J, Stokes J. Hazards of obesity: The Framingham experience. Acta Med Scand 1988; 723(suppl):23–36.

37. Hodsman GP, Johnson CL. Angiotensin converting enzyme inhibitors: drug interaction. Hypertension 1987; 5:1.

38. Holland BO, Nixon JV, Kuhnert LA. Diuretic induced ventricular ectopic activity. Am J Med 1980; 70:762–768.

39. Hollenberg NK, Swartz SL, Passan DR, Williams GH. Increased glomerular filtration rate after converting enzyme inhibition in essential hypertension. N Engl J Med 1979; 301:9–12.

40. Hollenberg NK, Meggs LG, Williams GH, Katz J, Garnic JD, Harrington DP. Sodium intake and renal responses to captopril in normal man and in essential hypertension. Kidney Int 1981; 20: 240–245.

41. Hollenberg NK. Initial therapy in hypertension: Quality of life considerations. J Hypertension 1987; 5(suppl 1):3.

42. Hollifield JW, Slaton PE. Thiazide diuretics, hypokalemia and cardiac arrhythmia. Acta Med Scand 1981; 647(suppl):67–73.

43. Hulley SB, Furberg CD, Gurland B. Systolic hypertension in the

elderly program: antihypertension efficiancy of chlorthalidone. Am J Cardiol 1985; 56:913–920.

44. Jenkins AC, Knill JR, Dreslinski GR. Captopril in the treatment of the elderly hypertensive patient. Arch Intern Med 1985; 145:2029–2031.

45. Jett GK. Captopril induced angioedema. Ann Emerg Med 1984; 13:489.

46. Kannel W, McGee D, Gordon T. A general cardiovascular risk profile: The Framingham Study. Am J Cardiol 1976; 38:46–52.

47. Kannel WB, Hjortland MC, McNamara M, Gordon T. Menopause and risk of cardiovascular disease: The Framingham Study. Ann Intern Med 1976; 85:447–452.

48. Kaplan NM. New approaches to the therapy of mild hypertension. Am J Cardiol 1983; 51:621–627.

49. Krebs R. Adverse reactions with calcium antagonists. Hypertension 1983; 5:125–129.

50. Kromer EP, Riegger AJ. Effects of long term angiotensin converting enzyme inhibition on myocardial hypertrophy in experimental aortic stenosis in the rat. Am J Cardiol 1988; 62:161–163.

51. LaCroix AZ, Wienphal J, White LR. Thiazide diuretics and the incidence of hip fractures. N Engl J Med 1990; 322:286–290.

52. Larochelle P, Gutkowska J, Schiffrin E, Kuchel O. Effect of enalapril on renin angiotensin converting enzyme, aldosterone and prostaglandins in patients with hypertension. Clin Invest Med 1985; 8:197–201.

53. Lerner DJ, Kannel WB. Patterns of coronary heart disease morbidity and mortality in the sexes: a 26-year follow up of the Framingham population. Am Heart J 1986; 111:383.

54. Leonetti G, Zanchetti A. Antihypertensive efficacy of nicardipine based treatment in patients of different age and in patients with isolated systolic hypertension. J Hypertension 1988 6(suppl 4): 655–657.

55. Levy D, Garrison RJ, Savage DD, Kannel WB, Castelli WP. Prognostic implications of echocardiographically determined left ventricular hypertrophy mass in the Framingham Heart Study. N Engl J Med 1990; 322:1561–1566.

56. Liebson PR. Clinical studies of drug reversal of hypertensive left ventricular hypertrophy. Am J Hypertension 1990; 3:512–517.

57. Linz W, Scholkens BA, Ganten D. Converting enzyme inhibition

specifically prevents the development and induces regression of cardiac hypertrophy in rats. Clin Exper Theory Prac 1989; A11(7):1325–1350.

58. Lund-Johansen P, Omvik PJ. Central hemodynamic changes of calcium antagonists at rest and during exercise in essential hypertension. Cardiovasc Pharmacol 1987; 10(suppl 1):S139–S148.

59. Matthews KA, Meilahn E, Kuller LH. Menopause and risk factors for coronary heart disease. N Engl J Med 1989; 321:641–646.

60. McAuley BJ, Schroeder JS. The use of diltiazem hydrochloride in cardiovascular disorders. Pharmacotherapy 1982; 2:121–131.

61. McKenna F, Davison AM. Renin and beta blockade: prorenin and aldosterone may explain the controversy. Clin Nephrol 1986; 25:149.

62. McMabon FG. Management of essential hypertension. Mount Kisco: Futura Publishing, 1984; 296–300, 407–410.

63. Meyers MG. Hydrochlorothiazide with or without amiloride for hypertension in the elderly. Ann Intern Med 1987; 147:1026–1030.

64. Middler S, Pak CYC, Murard F, Bartter F. Thiazide diuretics and calcium metabolism. Metabolism 1973; 22:139–146.

65. Morton JJ. ACE inhibitors and vascular structure and function. ACE Report 1991; 74:1–4.

66. Niarchos AP, Laragh JH. Renin dependency in isolated systolic hypertension. Am J Med 1984; 77:407–414.

67. Nobile-Orazio E, Sterzi R. Br Med J 1981; 283:948.

68. O'Mailia JJ, Sander GE, Giles TD. Nifedipine associated myocardial ischemia or infarction in the treatment of hypertensive urgencies. Ann Intern Med 1987; 107:185.

69. Opie LH. Calcium channel antagonists. Part II. Use and comparative efficacy in hypertension and supraventricular arrhythmias: Minor indication. Cardiovasc Drugs Ther 1988; 1:625.

70. Oren S. Immediate and short-term cardiovascular effect of Fosinopril, a new angiotensin converting enzyme inhibitor, in patients with essential hypertension. J Am Coll Cardiol 1991; 17:1183–1187.

71. Packer M, Lee WH, Yushak M, Medine N. Comparison of captopril and enalapril in patients with severe chronic heart failure. N Engl J Med 1986; 315:847–853.

72. Pickering TG, Harshfield G, Devereux R, Largh J. What is the role of ambulatory blood pressure monitoring in the management of hypertensive patients? Hypertension 1985; 7(2):171–177.

73. Pickering TG, O'Brien E. Second international consensus meeting on 24h ambulatory blood pressure measurement: consensus and conclusion. J Hypertension 1991; 9(suppl 8):2–6.

74. Pool PE, Massie BM, Venkataram AN. Diltiazem as a model therapy for systemic hypertension: a multicenter, randomized, placebo-controlled trial. Am J Cardiol 1986; 57:212–217.

75. Ray WA, Griffin MR, Downey W, Melton LJ. Long-term use of thiazide diuretics and risk of hip fracture. Lancet 1989; i:687–690.

76. Reams GP, Bauer JH. Long term effects of enalapril monotherapy and enalapril/hydrochlorothiazide combination therapy on blood pressure, renal function and body fluid composition. J Clin Hypertension 1986; 2:55–63.

77. Saner H, Brunner HR. Antihypertensive Wirksamkeit und Vertraglichkeit von Captopril. Ergebnisse einer Schweizer Feldstudie. Therapiewoche Schweiz 1988; 2:157.

78. Schmieder RE, Rockstroh JK, Messerli FH. Current recommendations for first line therapy of uncomplicated hypertension. In: Norwell, Andreucci VE, Fine LG, eds. International Yearbook of Nephrology. 1990:141–157.

79. Sernbo I, Johnell O. Consequences of hip fracture: a prospective study over 1 year. Osteoporosis Int 1993; 3:148–153.

80. Sever P, Beevers G, Bulpitt C, Lever A, Ramsay L, Reid J, Swales J. Management guidelines in essential hypertension: report of the second working party of the British Hypertension Society. Br Med J 1993; 306:983–986.

81. Stampfer MJ, Colditz GA, Willett WC. Postmenopausal estrogen therapy and cardiovascular disease: Ten-year follow up from the Nurses' Health Study. N Engl J Med 1991; 325:756–762.

82. Stokes J, Kannel WB, Wolf PA, D'Agostino RB, Cupples LA. Blood pressure as a risk factor for cardiovascular disease: The Framingham study—30 years of follow-up. Hypertension 1989; 13(suppl):113–118.

83. Transbol I, Christensen MS, Jensen GF, Christiansen C, Mac Nair P. Thiazide for the postponement of postmenopausal bone loss. Metabolism 1982; 31:383–386.

84. Todd PA. Enalapril: a review of its pharmakokinetic properties, and therapeutic use in hypertension and congestive heart failure. Drugs 1986; 31:198–248.

85. van Zwieten PA, Timmermans P, van Heiningen P. J Hypertension 1987; 5(suppl 4):21.

86. Vestal RE, Wood JJ, Shand DG. Reduced beta-adrenoreceptor sensitivity in the elderly. Clin Pharmacol 1979; 26:181–186.
87. Vidt G. Captopril. N Engl J Med 1982; 306:214–219.
88. Williams GF, Hollenberg NK. Accentuated vascular and endocrine response to SQ20881 in hypertension. N Engl J Med 1977; 297: 184–188.
89. Williams G, Donaldson RM. Nifedipine and nocturia. Lancet 1986; ii:738.
90. Wong LM, Zimmermann BG. Dependence of renal vasodilator effect of captopril on prevailing plasma renin level in the dog: influence of DOCA-salt treatment. Clin Sci 1982; 63:355–360.

14

Initiation and Monitoring of Hormone Replacement Therapy

Paul E. Belchetz

The General Infirmary at Leeds
Leeds, England

I. INTRODUCTION

Coronary artery disease is rare in premenopausal women compared with men of the same age. The situation changes after the menopause, especially in women who have undergone surgical oophorectomy (1–3). By the age of 65, cardiovascular disease is equally common in men and women. In the United States, 500,000 women die annually from cardiovascular disease, half due to coronary artery disease (4). There is now compelling evidence from observational studies that hormone replacement therapy of postmenopausal women greatly reduces the incidence of coronary artery disease. Retrospective evidence from case-control studies of women treated with estrogen—mostly unop-

posed conjugated equine estrogens—in the main indicate beneficial effects on the heart (Table 1) (5–14). The single exception
was a particularly small study in which the women enrolled were
unusually young and there was a strikingly high rate of smoking (7).

On reviewing prospective (but nonrandomized) trials of
estrogen therapy on postmenopausal women, there was again
largely a consensus indicating clear benefit in terms of coronary
disease, especially a lower rate of death (Table 2) (15–25). The
differences between the two Kaiser Permanente Walnut Creek
studies are interesting in that initially no benefit was shown
when nearly all the women were under 50 years old (16) whereas
7 years later fatal but not nonfatal cardiovascular disease was
reduced in women using estrogen (17). The apparent contradictory findings of the Framingham Study (19) and the Nurses'
Health Study (20) published sequentially in the *New England
Journal of Medicine* prompted much debate. The Framingham
Study was flawed by the use of angina as an endpoint, since this
correlates poorly with arteriographic evidence of coronary artery
disease. During the investigation of chest pain, normal coronary
arteries are found five times more commonly in women than men
(26). Furthermore, the Framingham Study did not collect details
of the dosage and duration of estrogen usage. Subsequent reanalysis of the Framingham data indicated a protective role for
estrogen in women under 60 (27).

These cumulative data have led to widespread acceptance
of the concept that estrogen use in postmenopausal women is
cardioprotective. Enthusiasts have proclaimed "benefit virtually
without risk if cardiovascular effects are considered" (28). A
meta-analysis performed to gain a quantitative estimate for the
size of benefit indicated a 40 to 50% reduction in the risk of
coronary heart disease due to the use of estrogen in postmenopausal women (29). Others have pointed out the selective bias
inherent in all observational trials in that those using estrogen
tend to share other factors favorable to their cardiac health, such
as high nonsmoker rates, attention to diet and weight, and compliance with medication as well as greater readiness to use

Table 1 Case-Control Studies of Hormone Replacement Therapy and Ischemic Heart Disease

Authors (Ref.)	Country	Data source	No. of cases	Relative risk	
				Ever-use	Current use
Rosenberg et al., 1976 (5)	U.S.	Interviews	336	Not reported	1.0
Pfeffer et al., 1978 (6)	U.S.	Pharmacy records	220	0.9	0.7
Jick et al., 1978 (7)	U.S.	Interviews	17	Not reported	4.2
Rosenberg et al., 1980 (8)	U.S.	Interviews	447	0.7 1.5	0.5 (30–44 yrs) 0.9 (45–59 yrs)
Ross et al., 1981 (9)	U.S.	Medical records	133	0.4 0.6	Not reported (living controls) Not reported (deceased controls)
Bain et al., 1981 (10)	U.S.	Mailed survey	123	0.8	0.7
Adam et al., 1981 (11)	U.K.	Doctor records	76	0.6	0.8
Szklo et al., 1984 (12)	U.S	Interviews	39	0.4	0.4
Croft and Hannaford, 1989 (13)	U.K.	Medical records		0.8	Not reported
Thompson et al., 1989 (14)	U.K.	Medical records	603	1.1	Not reported [strokes (244) and MI (359) analyzed together]

Source: Ref. 79.

Table 2 Cohort Studies of Estrogen Replacement Therapy and Ischemic Heart Disease

Authors (Ref.)	Country	Description of Cohort	Endpoint	No. of cases	Relative risk
Burch et al., 1974 (15)	U.S.	737 hysterectomized women	Fatal CHD	9	0.4
Petitti et al., 1979 (16)	U.S.	16,638 members of health plan	MI	26	1.2
Petitti et al., 1986 (17)	U.S.	16,638 members of health plan	Fatal MI		0.5
			Nonfatal MI		1.0
Hammond et al., 1979 (18)	U.S.	610 hypoestrogenic patients	CHD	58	0.3
Wilson et al., 1985 (19)	U.S.	1234 postmenopausal residents	CHD	116	1.9
			Fatal cardiovascular disease	48	1.9
Stampfer et al., 1985 (20)	U.S.	32,317 postmenopausal nurses	CHD: fatal and nonfatal	90	0.3 (current use) 0.5 (ever-use)
Hunt et al., 1987 (21)	U.K.	4544 postmenopausal British women	Fatal CHD	20	0.5
Bush et al., 1987 (22)	U.S.	2270 white women	Fatal CHD	50	0.4
Henderson et al., 1988 (23)	U.S.	8841 retirement community residents	Fatal MI	149	0.6
Criqui et al., 1988 (24)	U.S.	1868 residents of planned community	Fatal CHD	87	0.75
Stampfer et al., 1991 (25)	U.S.	48,470 postmenopausal nurses	CHD	45	0.5 (current use) 0.9 (former use)
			Fatal CD	21	0.5 (current use)
				55	0.8 (former use)

Source: Ref. 79.

medical services (30,31). Thus, current estimates of benefit may be overoptimistic. Many reviewers of the field have called for large-scale randomized prospective trials (30–35). Despite the daunting length and cost of such studies, at last action seems in prospect with the forthcoming multicenter Women's Health Initiative. Thus, although definitive epidemiological evidence is awaited, there can be little room for doubt that postmenopausal estrogen is beneficial for the heart.

II. HORMONE REGIMENS

A. Oral Estrogen

For many years, particularly in the United States, estrogen alone has been the mainstay of treatment. Estrogen ingested by mouth leads to hepatic sinusoidal concentrations that are four to five times greater than in peripheral blood (36). This is due to hepatic metabolism of the high levels arriving from the gut—the so-called first-pass effect. This also induces changes in hepatic metabolism—increasing synthesis and secretion of various hepatic proteins, including several coagulation factors and renin substrate, which could theoretically have adverse effects and changes in lipid apoproteins that may be beneficial. Synthetic 17α-alkylated estrogens such as ethinyl estradiol are not metabolized by 17β-estradiol dehydrogenase (37), which enhances their effect on the liver and potency, restricting their use to oral contraception rather than hormone replacement therapy.

In the United States, by far the most widely used estrogen is conjugated equine estrogen; it is the use of this that has yielded most of the long-term epidemiological data. It is a complex mixture derived from the urine of pregnant mares, with inevitable small variations that are appropriately handled to yield a standardized product. It comprises estrone (50%) and equilin (25%) plus small amounts of other equine estrogens conjugated as sulfate esters. These include equilenin, which has pronounced hepatic effects and prolonged half-life (38). In many parts of Europe, there is greater use of estradiol valerate and mixtures of estradiol, estrone, and estriol (39). Oral estradiol is largely converted to estrone in the gut mucosa and liver (40). Estrone itself is only a weak estrogen but is in reversible equilibrium with estradiol, providing a supply in the face of the almost complete loss of ovarian secretion of estradiol in postmenopausal women. Estriol, the third natural human estrogen, is not converted to estradiol and has considerably less biological activity. Only 1–2% of estriol taken by mouth reaches the circulation (36).

B. Parenteral Estrogen

Estrogen given parenterally evades hepatic first-pass metabolism. Of the several types of patch available, all supply estradiol for 3 to 4 days when applied to the skin (41). The earliest version employed a plastic reservoir containing the hormone in alcoholic solution from which it provided a steady supply transdermally on application to the skin. Subsequent types dispense with the reservoir since the estradiol is contained in the flat membrane stuck on the skin (42). Another transdermal preparation is estradiol gel rubbed into the skin. Solid pellets of estradiol may be implanted subcutaneously—these last many months, with quite wide variations in the rate of decline in levels of serum estradiol. Since some women experience "deficiency" symptoms while the serum concentration is still high (43), implantation should not be repeated until the estradiol level has fallen to values commensurate with the midfollicular phase of the menstrual cycle (400 pmol/L = 108 pg/ml). This is more cumbersome than the conventional practice of repeating implants routinely at 6-month intervals without prior checks of hormone levels. Careful study indicates that the mean interval for requiring repeat implants ranges from 9 months between first and second to 11 months thereafter (44). Women subjected to unmonitored higher-frequency implants frequently display estradiol levels five or more times higher than the abovementioned target range, sometimes with major physical symptoms, especially bloating, and potentially sufficient to enhance blood coagulability, in contrast to the situation with conventional estrogen replacement. Systemic delivery of estrogen can also be provided from vaginal pessaries or rings.

C. Combined Estrogen and Progestogen Preparations

The use of unopposed estrogen markedly increases the risk of endometrial hyperplasia and carcinoma (45,46), so the addition of a progestogen is routinely recommended in women with intact uteri (47–50). Natural progesterone may cause sleepiness and is poorly available by mouth, although micronized preparations are better absorbed (51), and use of progesterone pessaries or suppositories is also effective. Synthetic progestogens are effective orally and more generally used, although most have some androgenic activity, especially 19-nortestosterone derivatives such as norgestrel and norethindrone (noresthisterone) (36). C-21 pregnane derivatives such as medroxyprogesterone acetate, dydrogesterone, medrogestone, and megestrol acetate are very weak androgens. Recently introduced into use in combined oral contraceptives are progestogens with negligible androgenic properties—desogestrel, norgestimate, and gestodene—but these have yet to be used in routine hormone replacement regimens.

Continued menstruation is perceived as a major deterrent to the uptake or continued compliance with hormone replacement therapy. A further adverse factor is production of symptoms akin to premenstrual syndrome when a progestogen is added to the estrogen. Attempts is mitigate these symptoms include reducing the frequency of administration of progestogen to 12–14 days every 3 months, or using especially low doses of progestogen, e.g., two 350 μg tablets of norethindrone (norethisterone) for 12 days per cycle. An alternative approach has been to give estrogen and progestogen in combination continuously. This has been used extensively in Europe either as a synthetic steroid, Tibolone—which has both estrogenic and progestogenic properties, but also androgenic qualities in the one molecule—or as combinations of estradiol valerate and norethindrone. Both formulations are associated with at least a 40% incidence of breakthrough bleeding, especially in the first 6 months (52). As only the uterus needs progesterone, a progesterone-impregnated intrauterine device (Progestasert) has been developed to provide simply the local requirements, permitting the benefits of otherwise unopposed estrogen (53).

III. MECHANISMS MEDIATING HORMONAL INFLUENCES ON CARDIOVASCULAR DISEASE

In lieu of definitive evidence relating use of hormonal therapy to clinical outcome, several surrogate risk factors and pathophysiological mechanisms have been studied (54–56). The greatest emphasis has been placed on changes in serum lipids and lipoproteins, resulting in an enormous literature that has been the subject of several reviews. The use of oral estrogen raises the serum high-density lipoprotein (HDL) cholesterol concentrations, especially the HDL_2 subfraction, and reduces the low-density lipoprotein (LDL) cholesterol concentration, usually leading to a slight decrease in total cholesterol level. The favorable changes are the most widely cited explanations for the epidemiological data. Although oral estrogen raises serum triglyceride concentrations, this is not regarded as a major adverse effect (56). Parenterally administered estrogen (patch, gel, pessary, or implant) has little effect on HDL cholesterol; large amounts are needed to lower LDL cholesterol while triglycerides are virtually unchanged.

The conventional wisdom is that the rise in HDL cholesterol and the fall in LDL cholesterol brought about by estrogen are both attenuated by the addition of progestogen. This is reflected in reviews of the large number of studies involving many combinations of estrogens, progestogens, doses, and schedules. The androgenicity of the progestogen used is probably the major factor, but continuous estrogen–progestogen regimens have also been cast as having a more deleterious effect than conventional cyclical protocols. Recent studies suggest, by contrast, possible improvements in surrogate risk factors for cardiovascular disease in patients treated with estrogen plus progestogen (in the great majority, this is medroxyprogesterone acetate) compared with estrogen alone (57), and an apparently greater reduction in the risk of myocardial infarction in women on combined hormonal replacement therapy as opposed to estrogen only (58).

The Postmenopausal Estrogen/Progestin Interventions (PEPI) trial was a 3-year, multicenter, randomized, double-blind, placebo-controlled study involving 875 postmenopausal women aged 45 to 64 years assigned randomly to five equal groups. These were: 1) placebo, 2) conjugated equine estrogen (CEE) 0.625 mg daily, 3) CEE 0.625 mg plus medroxyprogesterone acetate (MPA) 10 mg for 12 days each month, 4) CEE 0.625 mg plus MPA 2.5 mg daily, 5) CEE 0.625 mg plus micronized progesterone 200 mg for 12 days each month. The results of this trial revealed that estrogen alone or combined with progestogen improved lipoproteins and lowered fibrinogen but there was no systemic effect on blood pressure or insulin levels (59).

A further area of potential benefit is the vasodilating property of estrogen (60,61), which may involve the generation of prostacyclin in vessel walls but might be reversed by progestogen (62).

IV. CONTRAINDICATIONS FOR THE USE OF ESTROGEN

With the passage of time, a previously formidable list of contraindications to estrogen use has been whittled down so that many women formerly excluded are now the prime candidates for it—this especially applies to the whole area of cardiovascular disease. Subsets thought to be particularly benefitted are those with adverse lipid profiles (although, of course, in severe cases additional treatment may be needed in addition to hormonal therapy to optimize the levels). Smokers are also thought to benefit rather than be at increased risk. Hypertension is not a contraindication for the use of estrogen; indeed, there is frequently some reduction in blood pressure. Idiosyncratic increases may be seen, however, so monitoring of blood pressure is mandatory and, where indicated, concomitant hypotensive drugs introduced or adjusted to ensure suitable reduction in arterial pressure.

One of the greatest areas of confusion is the persisting belief that hormonal replacement therapy predisposes to thromboembolic disease. This obsolete view has no foundation (63); indeed, recent studies suggest enhanced fibrinolytic activity, and a sharp distinction must be drawn from the situation with old-fashioned high-ethinyl-estradiol-dose oral contraceptive pills. The question continues to arise with patients who may have a thrombophilic tendency as judged by their personal medical history or family history. This has become more topical following the identification of the unsuspected high frequency of a point mutation in the factor V gene giving rise to resistance to the anticoagulant effect of activated protein C (APC resistance) (64). The heterozygote state not only enhances the likelihood of spontaneous venous thrombosis but is suggested to greatly increase the risk in oral contraceptive users (65). As yet, there is no evidence that the low dose of estrogen involved in estrogen replacement therapy acts in the same way. Indeed, the fact that APC resistance is present in 3–5% of Northern European populations (65,66), yet that there is no epidemiological association of hormone replacement therapy with increased risk of thrombosis, would suggest that this is not likely to be a relevant issue. There are at present no grounds for screens for APC resistance in women contemplating estrogen replacement.

Breast carcinoma is currently regarded as a contraindication for hormone replacement therapy on the basis of estrogen receptor positivity in many breast cancers and the epidemiological evidence that there is possibly a small increased incidence of breast cancer in women after at least 10 years of estrogen replacement (67–70). This dogma has been questioned (71,72), and careful studies are underway of women with breast carcinoma treated with estrogen because of severely debilitating menopausal symptoms. Nevertheless, it would seem prudent to avoid estrogen in these women if the sole indication is prophylaxis against cardiovascular disease.

A history of endometriosis is often regarded as a contraindication for estrogen therapy, although many women use it safely and painlessly. It may be wise to treat for 6 months with progestogen alone before adding estrogen in women who have undergone resection of endometriotic tissue with hysterectomy and bilateral oophorectomy (73). Rarely, ureteric involvement with endometriosis can lead to obstructive uropathy (74). Changes in composition of bile caused by estrogen may caution against its use in women with gallbladder disease (75). Catamenial migraine may return in postmenopausal women using hormonal replacement therapy (76).

V. MANAGEMENT OF HORMONAL THERAPY IN POSTMENOPAUSAL WOMEN

The information currently available must be regarded as incomplete, and the definitive answers expected of long-awaited prospective randomized trials—such as should emerge from the Women's Health Initiative—remain long distant (77). The ballpark is continually changing, not only with new studies providing clinical or laboratory data but also as different preparations become licensed—much variation in presenting patterns flows from differences in habit and availability in different countries.

Thus, the overwhelming preference for conjugated equine estrogen in North America based on long and safe experience with its use received a transient blow when allegations were made concerning the methods by which the pregnant mares' urine was collected. Fortunately, independent investigations by a Canadian animal rights organization refuted these charges. In Europe, more estradiol-containing preparations tend to be used (39,59). Transatlantic differences in progestogen usage may account in part for the more adverse reports regarding lipid profiles in women using combined estrogen–progestogen therapy in European studies, where there is a greater use of 19-nortestosterone derivatives such as norgestrel or norethindrone, whereas medroxyprogesterone acetate is by far the favored progestogen in the United States. A summary of preparations, including a num-

Table 3 Hormone Replacement Therapy Available in the U.K. (July 1995)

Type	Brand	Estrogen	Progestogen	Formulation	Strengths (of estrogen)	Bleed
Sequential combined therapy	Climagest	Estradiol	Norethindrone (Norethisterone)	Tabs	2 strengths (1, 2 mg)	M
	Cycloprogynova	Estradiol	Levonorgestrel	Tabs	2 strengths (1, 2 mg)	M
	Estracombi	Estradiol	Norethindrone (Norethisterone)	Patches	Single strength (50 μg)	M
	Estrapak	Estradiol	Norethindrone (Norethisterone)	Patches + tabs	Single strength (50 μg)	M
	Evorel-Pak	Estradiol	Norethindrone (Norethisterone)	Patches + tabs	Single strength (50 μg)	M
	Femoston 2/10	Estradiol	Dydrogesterone	Tabs	Single strength (2 mg)	M
	Femoston 2/20	Estradiol	Dydrogesterone	Tabs	Single strength (2 mg)	M
	Menophase	Mestranol	Norethindrone (Norethisterone)	Tabs	Single strength	M
	Nuvelle	Estradiol	Levonorgestrel	Tabs	Single strength (2 mg)	M
	Prempak-C	Conj. estrogens	Norgestrel	Tabs	2 strengths (0.625, 1.25 mg)	M
	Tridestra	Estradiol	Medroxyprogesterone	Tabs	Single strength (2 mg)	Q
	Trisequens	Estradiol/estriol	Norenthindrone (Norethisterone)	Tabs	2 strengths	M
Continuous combined therapy	Klofem	Estradiol	Norethindrone (Norethisterone)	Tabs	Single strength (2 mg)	X

	Product	Ingredient	Form	Strength	
Gonadomimetic	Livial		Tabs	Single strength	X
Unopposed estrogen	Climaval	Estradiol	Tabs	2 strengths (1, 2 mg)	
	Estraderm	Estradiol	Patches	3 strengths (25, 50, 100 µg)	
	Evorel	Estradiol	Patches	4 strengths (25, 50, 75, 100 µg)	
	Fematrix	Estradiol	Patches	Single strength (80 µg)	
	Harmogen	Estrone	Tabs	Single strength (0.93 mg)	
	Hormonin	Estriol/estradiol/estrone	Tabs	Single strength	
	Oestrogel	Estradiol	Gel	Single strength (1.5 mg)	
	Premarin	Conj. estrogens	Tabs	2 strengths (0.625, 1.25 mg)	
	Progynova	Estradiol	Tabs	2 strengths (1, 2 mg)	
	Zumenon	Estradiol	Tabs	Single strength (2 mg)	
		Estradiol	Pellets	3 strengths (25, 50, 100 mg)	
Adjunctive progestogen	Duphaston HRT	Dydrogesterone	Tabs	Single strength	
	Micronor HRT	Norethindrone (Norethisterone)	Tabs	Single strength	

M = monthly; Q = quarterly; X = no bleeding.

Source: Adapted from Monthly Index of Medical Specialities, September 1995, by permission of Haymarket Medical Ltd.

Table 4 Hormone Replacement Therapy Using Unopposed Estrogen

Candidates	First-line therapy	Alternative therapy	Duration	Precautions
1. Hysterectomized women 2. Women with intact uteri Strictly limit to those with: a. Severe persistent menopausal symptoms but unable to tolerate progestogens b. High cardiovascular risk due to markedly adverse cholesterol profile (raised LDL:HDL ratio)	Oral therapy, e.g., Premarin 0.625 mg or estradiol valerate 2 mg daily (continuous, not cyclical therapy)	Parenteral therapy, e.g., Estraderm TTS patches—use if intolerance of oral preparations, in hypertensive patients (but control blood pressure), past history of venous thromboembolism, stable liver disease. If skin reactions occur, consider estradiol implants.	1. Menopausal symptoms: 5 years—if symptoms recur, further 5 years or indefinitely if necessary. 2. Cardiovascular disease: lifelong—current use provides maximum benefit. 3. Osteoporosis: lifelong optimal but 10 years' use probably defers rise in hip fracture from 70 to 80 years. After 80, calcium supplements, calcitonin, or vitamin D may be preferable.	1. Breast cancer: slight increase observed after 10 years' use, thereafter mammograms at baseline and 18-month to 2-year intervals while on treatment. 2. Endometrial surveillance: mandatory if used in women with intact uteri, repeat 2-yearly, indefinitely even if therapy ceases.

Source: Ref. 79.

Table 5 Hormone Replacement Therapy Using Combination Estrogen–Progestogen

Candidates	First-line therapy	Alternative therapy	Duration	Precautions
1. Most women with intact uteri 2. Can be considered in women who have undergone hysterectomy and oophorectomy for endometriosis or stage I or II carcinoma of endometrium	Continuous oral estrogen, e.g., Premarin 0.625 mg or estradiol valerate 2 mg, plus 10–12 days/cycle low-dose progestogen, e.g., medroxyprogesterone acetate, norethindrone, or norgestrel	Second-line therapy: transdermal estrogen patches with oral (or, more recently, transdermal) progestogen for 10–12 days/cycle Third-line therapy: continuous combined estrogen–progestogen or tibolone (Livial) to avoid menstrual activity	1. Menopausal symptoms: as for unopposed estrogen 2. Cardiovascular disease: no current evidence that combination therapy is protective (or overtly harmful compared with no treatment), therefore not used as prophylaxis against ischemic heart disease 3. Osteoporosis: as for unopposed estrogen	1. Breast cancer: as for unopposed estrogen 2. Endometrial cancer: gynecologic examination prior to therapy; endometrial surveillance unnecessary in absence of unscheduled bleeding if full progestogen (10–12 days/cycle) used 3. Cardiovascular disease: monitor blood pressure 3-monthly in first year; if normotensive, annually thereafter. Hypertension, closely monitored and well controlled, is not a contraindication. Combination therapy contraindicated with hyperlipidemia or established ischemic heart disease.

Source: Ref. 79.

ber that have very recently received their license in the United Kingdom, is given in Table 3.

It remains necessary to acknowledge that any recommendations, even in a consensus view such as appeared in the American College of Physicians guidelines (78), are simply best attempts to interpret the currently available information. What appears in Tables 4 and 5 is therefore an admittedly personal and subjective view prepared by the author for a review that appeared in 1994 (79). Although discernible shifts in emphasis have occurred subsequently, it is felt prudent and conservative to maintain this view at present since, for example, the data indicating greater safety with conjugated equine estrogen and MPA than estrogen alone may not be repeated when other regimens are critically evaluated.

REFERENCES

1. Kannel WB, Hjortland MC, McNamara PM, Gordon T. Menopause and risk of cardiovascular disease: The Framingham Study. Ann Intern Med 1976; 85:447–452.
2. Colditz GA, Willett WC, Stampfer MJ, et al. Menopause and the risk of coronary heart disease in women. N Engl J Med 1987; 316:1105–1110.
3. Wuest JH, Dry TJ, Edwards JE. The degree of coronary atherosclerosis in bilaterally oophorectomized women. Circulation 1953; 7:801–809.
4. Heart and Stroke Facts. Dallas: American Heart Foundation, 1992.
5. Rosenberg L, Armstrong B, Jick H. Myocardial infarction and estrogen therapy in postmenopausal women. N Engl J Med 1976; 294:1256–1259.
6. Pfeffer RI, Whipple GH, Kurosaki TT, Chapman JM, Coronary risk and estrogen use in postmenopausal women. Am J Epidemiol 1978; 107:479–497.
7. Jick H, Dinan B, Rothman KJ. Noncontraceptive estrogens and nonfatal myocardial infarction. JAMA 1978; 239:1407–1409.
8. Rosenberg L, Slone D, Shapiro S, et al. Noncontraceptive estrogens and myocardial infarction in young women. JAMA 1980; 244:339–342.
9. Ross RK, Paganini-Hill A, Mack TM, et al. Menopausal oestrogen

therapy and protection from death from ischaemic heart disease. Lancet 1981; i:858–860.

10. Bain C, Willett W, Hennekens CH, et al. Use of postmenopausal hormones and risk of myocardial infarction. Circulation 1981; 64:42–46.

11. Adam S, Williams V, Vessey MP. Cardiovascular disease and hormone replacement treatment: a pilot case-control study. Br Med J 1981; 282:1277–1278.

12. Szklo M, Tonascia J, Gordis L, Bloom I. Estrogen use and myocardial infarction risk: a case-control study. Prev Med 1984; 13: 510–516.

13. Croft P, Hannaford PC. Risk factors for acute myocardial infarction in women: evidence from the Royal College of General Practitioners' oral contraception study. Br Med J 1989; 298:165–168.

14. Thompson SG, Meade TW, Greenberg G. The use of hormonal replacement therapy and the risk of stroke and myocardial infarction in women. J. Epidemiol Community Health 1989; 43: 173–178.

15. Burch JC, Byrd BF Jr, Vaughn WK. The effects of long term estrogen in hysterectomized women. Am J Obstet Gynecol 1974; 118:778–782.

16. Petitti DB, Wingerd J, Pellegrin F, Ramcharan S. Risk of vascular disease in women: Smoking, oral contraceptives, non-contraceptive estrogens, and other factors. JAMA 1979; 242:1150–1154.

17. Petitti DB, Perlman JA, Sidney S. Postmenopausal estrogen use and heart disease. N Engl J Med 1986; 315:131–132.

18. Hammond CB, Jelovsek FR, Lee KL, et al. Effects of long-term estrogen replacement therapy. 1. Metabolic effects. Am J Obstet Gynecol 1979; 133:525–536.

19. Wilson PWF, Garrison RJ, Castelli WP. Postmenopausal estrogen use, cigarette smoking, and cardiovascular morbidity in women over 50: The Framingham Study. N Engl J Med 1985; 313:1038–1043.

20. Stampfer MJ, Willett WC, Colditz GA, et al. A prospective study of postmenopausal estrogen therapy and coronary heart disease. N Engl J Med 1985; 313:1044–1049.

21. Hunt K, Vessey M, McPherson K, Coleman M. Long-term surveillance of mortality and cancer incidence in women receiving hormone replacement therapy. Br J Obstet Gynaecol 1987; 94:620–635.

22. Bush TL, Barrett-Connor E, Cowan LD, et al. Cardiovascular mortality and noncontraceptive use of estrogen in women: results from

the Lipid Research Clinics Program Follow-up Study. Circulation 1987; 75:1102–1109.

23. Henderson BE, Paganini-Hill A, Ross RK. Estrogen replacement therapy and protection from acute myocardial infarction. Am J Obstet Gynecol 1988; 159:312–317.

24. Criqui MH, Suarez L, Barrett-Connor E, et al. Postmenopausal estrogen use and mortality: Results from a prospective study in a defined, homogeneous community. Am J Epidemiol 1988; 128: 606–614.

25. Stampfer MJ, Colditz GA, Willett WC, et al. Postmenopausal estrogen therapy and cardiovascular disease: Ten-year follow-up from the nurses' health study. N Engl J Med 1991; 325:756–762.

26. Sullivan AK, Holdright DR, Wright CA, Sparrow JL, Cunningham D, Fox KM. Chest pain in women: clinical investigative and prognostic features. Br Med J 1994; 308:883–886.

27. Eaker ED, Castelli WP. Coronary heart disease and its risk factors among women in the Framingham Study. In: Eaker ED, Packard B, Wenger NK, Clarkson TB, Tyroler HA, eds. Coronary Disease in Women. New York: Haymarket Doyma, 1987:122–132.

28. Hillner BE, Hollenberg JP, Pauker SG. Postmenopausal estrogens in prevention of osteoporosis: Benefit virtually without risk if cardiovascular effects are considered. Am J Med 1986; 80:1115–1127.

29. Stampfer MJ, Colditz GA. Estrogen replacement therapy and coronary heart disease: a quantitative assessment of the epidemiologic evidence. Prev Med 1991; 20:47–63.

30. Barrett-Connor E. Postmenopausal estrogen and prevention bias. Ann Intern Med 1991; 115:455–456.

31. Vandenbroucke JP. Postmenopausal oestrogen and cardioprotection. Lancet 1991; 337:833–834.

32. Ernster VL, Bush TL, Huggins GR, et al. Benefits and risks of menopausal estrogen and/or progestin hormone use. Prev Med 1988; 17:201–223.

33. Moon TE. Estrogens and disease prevention. Arch Intern Med 1991; 151:17–18.

34. Goldman L, Tosteson ANA. Uncertainty about postmenopausal estrogen: Time for action, not debate. N Engl J Med 1991; 325: 800–802.

35. Beaglehole R. Oestrogens and cardiovascular disease: Postmenopausal oestrogens seem to reduce coronary heart disease. Br Med J 1988; 297:571–572.

36. Kuhl H. Pharmacokinetics of oestrogens and progestogens. Maturitas 1990; 12:171–197.

37. von Schoultz B. Potency of different oestrogen preparations. In: Studd JWW, Whitehead MI, eds. The Menopause. Oxford: Blackwell Scientific Publications, 1988:130–137.

38. Bhavnani BR, Woolever CA, Benoit H, Wong T. Pharmacodynamics of equilin and equilin sulfate in normal postmenopausal women and men. J Clin Endocrinol Metab 1983; 56:1048–1056.

39. Persson I, Adami II-O, Lindberg BS, et al. Practice and patterns of estrogen treatment in climacteric women in a Swedish population. Acta Obstet Gynecol Scand 1983; 62:289–296.

40. Hutton JD, Jacobs HS, James VHT. Steroid endocrinology after the menopause: a review. J R Soc Med 1979; 72:835–841.

41. Powers MS, Schenkel L, Darley PE, et al. Pharmacokinetics and pharmacodynamics of transdermal dosage forms of 17β-estradiol: comparison with conventional oral estrogens used for hormone replacement. Am J Obstet Gynecol 1985; 152:1099–1106.

42. McCarthy T, Dramusic V, Ratnam S. Use of two types of estradiol-releasing skin patches for menopausal women in a tropical climate. Am J Obstet Gynecol 1992; 166:2005–2010.

43. Gangar K, Cust M, Whitehead MI. Symptoms of oestrogen deficiency associated with supraphysiological plasma oestradiol concentrations in women with oestradiol implants. Br Med J 1989; 299:601–602.

44. Buckler HM, Kalsi PK, Cantrill JA, Anderson DC. An audit of oestradiol levels and implant frequency in women undergoing subcutaneous implant therapy. Clin Endocrinol 1995; 42:445–450.

45. Smith DC, Prentice R, Thompson DJ, Herrmann WL. Association of exogenous estrogens and endometrial carcinoma. N Engl J Med 1975; 293:1164–1167.

46. Ziel HK, Finkle WD. Increased risk of endometrial carcinoma among users of conjugated estrogens. N Engl J Med 1975; 293: 1167–1170.

47. Gambrell RD Jr. Prevention of endometrial cancer with progestogens. Maturitas 1986; 8:159–168.

48. Persson I, Adami HO, Bergkvist L, et al. Risk of endometrial cancer after treatment with oestrogens alone or in conjunction with progestogens: results of a prospective study. Br Med J 1989; 298:147–151.

49. Voight LF, Weiss NS, Chu J, et al. Progestagen supplementation of exogenous oestrogens and risk of endometrial cancer. Lancet 1991; 338:274–277.

50. Whitehead MI, Townsend PT, Pryse-Davies J, et al. Effects of estrogens and progestins on the biochemistry and morphology of the postmenopausal endometrium. N Engl J Med 1981; 305:1599–1605.
51. Arafat ES, Hargrave JT, Maxson WS, et al. Sedative and hypnotic effects of oral administration of micronized progesterone may be mediated through its metabolites. Am J Obstet Gynecol 1988; 159:1203–1209.
52. Christiansen C, Riis BJ. Five years with continuous combined oestrogen/progestogen therapy: Effects on calcium metabolism, lipoproteins and bleeding patterns. Br J Obstet Gynaeol 1990; 97:1087–1092.
53. Shoupe D, Meme D, Mezrow G, Lobo RA. Prevention of endometrial hyperplasia in postmenopausal women with intrauterine progesterone. N Engl J Med 1991; 235:1811–1812.
54. Rijpkema AHM, van der Sanden AA, Ruijs AHC. Effects of postmenopausal oestrogen-progestogen replacement therapy on serum lipids and lipoproteins: a review. Maturitas 1990; 12:259–285.
55. Lobo RA. Effects of hormonal replacement on lipids and lipoproteins in postmenopausal women. J Clin Endocrinol Metab 1991; 73:925–930.
56. Walsh BW, Schiff I, Rosner B, et al. Effects of postmenopausal estrogen replacement on the concentrations and metabolism of plasma lipoproteins. N Engl J Med 1991; 325:1196–1204.
57. Nabulsi A, Folsom AR, White A, et al. Association of hormone-replacement therapy with various cardiovascular factors in postmenopausal women. N Engl J Med 1993; 328:1069–1075.
58. Falkeborn M, Persson I, Adami H-O, et al. The risk of acute myocardial infarction after oestrogen and oestrogen-progestogen replacement. Br J Obstet Gynaecol 1992; 99:821–828.
59. The writing group for the PEPI trial. Effects of estrogen or estrogen/progestin regimens on heart disease risk factors in postmenopausal women. JAMA 1995; 273:199–208.
60. Sarrel PM. Ovarian hormones and the circulation. Maturitas 1990; 12:287–298.
61. Gangar KF, Vyas S, Whitehead M, et al. Pulsatility index in internal carotid artery in relation to transdermal oestradiol and time since menopause. Lancet 1991; 338:839–842.
62. Wren BG. Hypertension and thrombosis with postmenopausal oestrogen therapy. In: Studd JWW, Whitehead MI, eds. The Menopause. Oxford: Blackwell Scientific Publications, 1988: 181–189.

63. Meade TW. Oestrogen and thrombosis. In: Drife JO, Studd JWW, eds. HRT and Osteoporosis. London: Springer-Verlag, 1990; 223–233.

64. Bertina RM, Koelman RPC, Koster T. Mutation in blood coagulation factor V associated with resistance to activated protein C. Nature 1994; 369:1515–1516.

65. Vandenbroucke JP, Koster T, Briët E, Reitsma PH, Bertina RM, Rosendaal FR. Increased risk of venous thrombosis in oral-contraceptive users who are carriers of factor V Leiden mutation. Lancet 1994; 344:1453–1457.

66. Svensson PJ, Dahlbäck B. Resistance to activated protein C as a basis for venous thrombosis. N Engl J Med 1994; 330:517–522.

67. Bergkvist L, Adami H-O, Persson I, et al. The risk of breast cancer after estrogen and estrogen-progestin replacement. N Engl J Med 1989; 321:293–297.

68. Colditz GA, Stampfer MJ, Willett WC, et al. Prospective study of estrogen replacement therapy and risk of breast cancer in postmenopausal women. JAMA 1990; 264:2648–2653.

69. Colditz GA, Stampfer MJ, Willett WC, et al. Postmenopausal hormone use and risk of breast cancer: 12-year follow-up of the Nurses' health study. In: Mann RD, ed. Hormone Replacement Therapy and Breast Cancer Risk. Carnforth: Parthenon Publishing Group, 1992:63–77.

70. Steinberg KK, Thacker SB, Smith SJ, et al. A meta-analysis of the effect of estrogen replacement therapy on the risk of breast cancer. JAMA 1991; 265:1985–1990.

71. Stoll BA, Parbhoo S. Treatment of menopausal symptoms in breast cancer patients. Lancet 1988; i:1278–1279.

72. Creasman WT. Estrogen replacement therapy: is previously treated cancer a contraindication? Obstet Gynecol 1991; 77:308–312.

73. Varner RE. Hormone replacement therapy. In: Shingleton HM, Hurt WG. Postreproductive Gynecology. New York: Churchill-Livingstone, 1990:143–169.

74. Goodman HM, Kredentser D, Deligdisch L. Postmenopausal endometriosis associated with hormone replacement therapy: A case report. J Reprod Med 1989; 34:231–233.

75. The Boston Collaborative Drug Surveillance Program. Surgically confirmed gall bladder disease, venous thromboembolism, and breast tumors in relation to postmenopausal estrogen therapy. N Engl J Med 1974; 290:15–18.

76. Edelson RN. Menstrual migraine and other hormonal aspects of migraine. Headache 1985; 25:376–379.
77. Rich-Edwards JW, Manson JE, Hennekens CH, Buring JE. The primary prevention of coronary heart disease in women. N Engl J Med 1995; 332:1758–1766.
78. American College of Physicians. Guidelines for counselling post-menopausal women about preventive hormone therapy. Ann Intern Med 1992; 117:1038–1041.
79. Belchetz PE. Hormonal treatment of postmenopausal women. N Engl J Med 1994; 330:1062–1071.

INDEX